Caregiver Triumphant

How to overcome stress and thrive in your role as a family caregiver

Vena Stewart-Semprie

Caregiver Triumphant:
How to overcome stress and thrive in your role as a family caregiver

Copyright © 2016 Vena Stewart-Semprie
All rights reserved

Cover design & photo by Hans Clough. HansClough.com

Some material in this book taken from or adapted from material found at plrplr.com
See http://plrplr.com/private-label-rights/

Dedicated with love, to caregivers, who courageously endure enormous challenges and self sacrifice, often times at the peril of your own needs, to love yourself and take care of your overall health first, and as a result, be better able to help the people you love.

Table of Contents

What this book will do for you   7

My life as a caregiver   11

Acceptance   22

Coping with caregiver stress   27

Caregiver depression   37

How to avoid caregiver burnout   42

How to overcome fear & worry   47

How to use the power of the universe to improve your health   50

A 10-step guide to create your own anesthesia to numb your pain   54

Making changes   61

The dangers of caregiver denial   63

Blessings come from suffering   68

How to manage guilt so guilt serves you not imprisons you   72

The freedom of forgiving others   76

Positive thinking and a new direction   83

Your identity   87

Do you really know what you want to be in life?   91

Setting goals   95

Visualization   100

Successful action	103
Commitment	109
The winner's walk	113
Resources for caregivers	115
Books	115
Websites	127
Facebook	151
Google+ communities	154
In recognition of World MS Day	156
About the author	158

If you really want to live, we'd better start at once to try;
If we don't it doesn't matter, we'd better start to die.
W. H. Auden

What this book will do for you

I write this book believing my experiences will bring hope and help to you if you are caring for family members with chronic illness.

For the past twenty-three years, I've been caring for my husband who has multiple sclerosis. (We've been married for forty-seven years.) I tell you openly it is the most difficult experience I ever lived. Had I known then what I know now, I would have approached this chronic illness in my family in a very different way. But twenty-three years ago, the information and support that is now available was only a work in progress. However, living through the difficulties I have overcome has enabled me to speak with authority so you can be better informed, and make better decisions.

Being a caregiver can be immensely rewarding. In addition to being there for someone you love, care giving can enhance family closeness, and offer emotional, psychological and spiritual rewards. Many caregivers experience a feeling of personal satisfaction by performing their role well, and their own confidence can grow as a result. Care giving is a complex role, and the interpersonal relationships, scheduling, monitoring medications and taking care of financial obligations can ward off cognitive decline.

However, care giving can present enormous challenges. Caregivers are at increased risk for depression, anxiety, depressed immune function and even hospitalization. Care giving places a burden on your health. This act of love also carries a financial burden. Caregivers stand to forfeit up to $650,000 or more in lost wages, pension and social security. Add to that the personal costs to your well being, as the demands of care giving leave you less time for your family and friends. You may find yourself giving up vacations, hobbies, and social activities. Solo care giving challenges your ability to nurture yourself and others.

Caregivers are competent people who feel that they should be able to fulfill this role. Yet, many soon find themselves unprepared and ill-equipped to manage the sometimes daunting tasks, such as managing a complex medical regimen or remodeling a house so it is wheel-chair accessible or even finding someone to stay with their loved ones so they can go out to a movie without worrying their relatives will fall on the way to the fridge.

Instead of reaching out, many caregivers become isolated. Many who assume the care giving role fit the profile of the giving family member and don't want to trouble others with their problems. Some fear the consequences of disclosing their new demands to coworkers or employers. Caregivers are further challenged by the cultural conspiracy of silence. Our youth-centered society turns a blind eye to the unpleasant and inevitable reality that all of us age and die. This leaves both caregivers and care recipients unprepared. Look no further than the path of Hurricane Katrina to witness the consequences of a lack of planning.

In view of these challenges, let's take care giving out from behind closed doors. For your sake and for the sake of those who count on you, please get the help you need.

Even if you are not currently a caregiver, you should have a plan in place in case care giving becomes a reality in your life.

What can you do? Start talking about "what if" and make a plan.

Start with yourself. What will happen to you and your family if you become disabled or die unexpectedly? Do you have disability insurance? Do you have a will? Do you have a living will, and have you identified the person who will make the medical choices you would make if you are not in the position to do so?

In addition, approach healthy family members. You can say, "I hope that you live many happy years in which you enjoy all of the pleasures you worked so hard to create." Have you thought about what would happen to you in the event that you cannot live independently any more? What would happen if some medical event befalls you? Who would make your medical choices?

Care giving is here to stay; it's not going anywhere. Open up your hearts and your minds and let the sun shine in. Get organized and prepare to face the challenges.

After reading this book, you will be in a position to make life easier on yourself and your family. Reach out to family, friends, medical professionals, and the resources identified in this book. You'll need all the help and support that's available to you. Most importantly, the onus is on you to take care of yourself first.

Lord, make me an instrument of Your peace.
Where there is hatred let me sow love;
Where there is injury, pardon;
Where there is doubt, faith;
Where there is despair, hope;
Where there is darkness, light; and
Where there is sadness, joy.
Saint Francis of Assisi

My life as a caregiver

I hoped it was only for a season

Care giving for me became a reality with the birth of my first son in 1969. At age 26, I had no idea how to care for a new-born baby. I was a new immigrant with no relatives here. I was married for one year. After spending a week at Mount Sinai hospital both baby and I were discharged, sent home. Reality was now happening!

This little angel, a beautiful bundle of joy, was fully dependent on me for everything. I had to learn fast. With the help of my husband, I grew accustomed to caring for our baby and eventually became quite good at it. Over the next ten years I gave birth to three more babies and continued in my role of care giving eagerly looking forward to the day when my responsibility of care giving would be no more.

My husband's diagnosis

Unfortunately, that did not happen. When my daughter was thirteen years old, my husband was diagnosed with chronic progressive multiple sclerosis (MS).

Little did I know that this disease would change our lives forever. A new journey of care giving began, and I am his care-giver to this present day.

What is MS? Multiple sclerosis (MS) is an inflammatory disease of the central nervous system (CNS)—that's the brain and spinal cord. Predominantly, it is a disease of the "white matter" tissue. The white matter is made up of nerve fibers which are responsible for transmitting communication signals both internally within the CNS and between the CNS and the nerves supplying the rest of the body.

MS was unknown to me. I had no idea what this monstrous disease was until the universe threw me this tremendous curve ball in the prime of life and I had to deal with it head on or bail on my family. The latter was not an option; I decided *I am not going anywhere.*

First, I had to learn about this debilitating disease in order to care for my husband, so I started my research in the library and on the Internet. Whatever knowledge I gained about MS would enable me to better understand the disease and how it might affect my husband as well as my entire family.

Being totally inexperienced and unprepared facing my new reality, the MS challenge, I decided to put a plan in place so my husband would live as normal a life as possible for as long as it was possible.

I focused on diet, exercise, rest and relaxation. My husband's diet was comprised of simple, healthy meals that included fruit, vegetables, fish, meat in moderation, beans, lots of greens and so on. My family ate the same balanced meals and incorporated exercise as a part of the healing process.

Fully cognizant of my added responsibilities I knew I must pay special attention to myself keeping in mind that I have to not only care for my husband but for my children and myself.

My husband's career

My husband was a detective employed with Toronto Police Service when he was diagnosed with MS in 1992, approximately 23 years into his career.

He retired from the Police Service in 1996, took a year off, and then started his own consulting agency, National Pardon Agency in 1997, which he operates at present.

The consulting agency gives him a reason to wake up each morning aware that he is still able to help out people that have/had issues with law enforcement. Ironically, these are some of the same people he dealt with back in his day as a detective. Now he helps rehabilitate these past offenders, empowering them to merge back into society as contributing members. This role is definitely an important factor that has prolonged his mobility. He is determined to carry on for as long as he possibly can and that quality is to be admired. Keeping active plays a major role in him being able to mobilize although with much difficulty.

Making mistakes

Care giving is not easy. Our new reality is living in a constant state of stress on a daily basis. My life's experience has been quite a journey, and I made enormous mistakes due to not knowing what I should have known. That said, these mistakes have enabled me to find my voice and to bring awareness to the world from my personal experience. Looking back, if only I knew then what I know now, I would take a completely different approach in handling the curve ball I was thrown. On a positive note, I now have the opportunity to share the difficulties I am experiencing and I trust we can all learn from other peoples' experiences so the outcome of our decisions will be less painful.

Although I empathize with my husband, I can never truly know what he feels or thinks about living with this debilitating condition. For the most part he internalizes his feelings, he keeps it all to himself. Truth be said, I do not know exactly what's going on in his head, however, I know enough to hear and to see the frustration he expresses from time to time not being able to lift his leg and mobilize as he once did.

I see the emotional anguish he suffers, often shedding tears. It is quite difficult for him to talk about his condition; he does not like to go there and it takes two to have a dialogue; however, whenever he brings up the topic I am always ready to listen.

Our failure to communicate meant that I had no way of judging his capabilities, nor did I have any way of setting healthy boundaries. As a result, I took on responsibilities that I wasn't prepared to handle, and lived with stress that I didn't need to carry. As these realities became clear to me over time, I struggled with a deep feeling of frustration and discontent. I saw that some elements of our relationship were not healthy, and that caused suffering no doubt for both of us.

Probably every married person would like to change his or her spouse. But spouses don't change because we want them to. They change if and when they want to. Meanwhile, we need to deal with our own feelings, our own issues, our own struggles.

The Serenity Prayer

For me, so much of my journey has been centered around learning to accept the things I cannot change. Maybe that's why the Serenity Prayer has become such an important part of my life.

> *God give me the serenity to accept the things I cannot change,*
> *the courage to change the things I can,*
> *and the wisdom to know the difference.*
> Reinhold Niebuhr
> The Serenity Prayer

Each day I pray the Serenity Prayer. Why? Life can be so daunting that I need to be grounded. If I entertain all the crazy random thoughts that go through my mind I would probably run amok, and, that's not a place where I want to be. Instead, I chose to tackle those crazy random thoughts and somehow I manage to find a positive out of every negative. I consider each challenge a learning opportunity and that positive attitude affords me the courage to cope from day to day.

Maturity and life's experience has given me the opportunity to learn, to grow, and to develop into a truly calm, serene human being. This transformation did not happen overnight; it came through many years of living real life's experiences. Giving blood, sweat and tears in working through enormous struggles and challenges, emerging triumphant in the end. Through the grace of God Almighty I am still standing in my role of caregiver.

As caregiver for my husband, my life is anything but normal. Life for me is truly difficult. There are good days and there are bad days for both of us. After all, we are only human. The beauty is that I never allow myself to stay down for long. I pick myself up, pray the serenity prayer, dust off and carry on. Life goes on with or without you.

Learning to accept

In spite of these challenges I have learned to accept the things I cannot change, to live in the moment and to focus on life's blessings. I do this through prayer and meditation reminding myself to accept the things I cannot change, for acceptance in any situation is the key to coping. The situation is what it is, and life goes on.

If I wake up in the morning and allow my thoughts to run rampant, I can most likely end up in a rut all day, or, I can feel truly accomplished at the end of the day. It all depends on how I manage my thoughts—I can succumb, or I can control. As soon as I remind myself to accept the things I cannot change, it all falls right back in place.

The same is true for feelings. Sometimes as I go through my struggles and challenges I feel the weight of the world resting on my shoulders. That's not a good place to be. I cannot allow those feelings to linger. I take control of my mind right away. I find something to laugh about. I laugh at myself. I sing something uplifting. I say a prayer.

Working out and massage

One of my favorite activities is working out at the gym. I am fortunate to have a personal trainer (my son) and train on a regular basis. (Working out is an option that's available to almost every caregiver—with or without a personal trainer. If you are part of a gym, usually staff members are willing to provide a great deal of extra help for free.) My gym activity enables me to cater to my mental and physical health providing clarity of mind and in strengthening my core through pilates training so I can take care of others.

Once a month, I have a full-body massage. These are some simple things I do that help to keep me mentally and physically fit and make me happy, knowing that I am doing something for me. You can do them too! Look good and feel good about yourself.

Cultivating my spiritual health

I get through each day with a positive attitude, reminding myself that there must be a reason why I am in this situation. Because I do not understand why I am where I am, I always ask this question to myself, *What would Jesus do given my situation?* I am convinced that my faith in God the Father, God the Son and God the Holy Spirit guides me in becoming the person I am today.

I incorporate simple things I enjoy in my daily life. I focus on me first; I try to take a daily walk and attend church when possible. Knowing that I've done something for me makes it easier to give and take care of others.

I attend church on Sundays and pay attention to the homily. (I am Catholic.) I find inspiration and comfort being in the presence of God listening to the readings and enjoying the beautiful hymns sung by choir and the congregation. To be a part of such wonderful experience, receiving the body and blood of our Lord and Savior, Jesus Christ through the sacred sacrament, energizes and brings me a new perspective for the week ahead. I am confident that divine intervention is what keeps me going as I could not journey alone.

I pray frequently and have an ongoing conversation with God Almighty, my Maker. In the end there's a feeling of relief, being able to release the emotions within, knowing that my God is taking care of me.

I read books that keep me motivated and I make a concerted effort to stay grounded. Believe me, it is a constant work in progress, it takes energy, focus and most importantly ongoing prayer.

My favorite word is beautiful. I look to find beauty in every-thing and always manage to find the positive in a negative.

My resolve in my journey as a caregiver is this: I will do the best I can where I am with what I have. I will love, care and give unconditionally, for, I love myself and can love anyone and anything. I will find the positive out of every negative and live in the moment. I will continue to thank God, the Father Almighty, for the precious gift of life and for the very many blessings bestowed upon me.

I look at myself as someone blessed and special. My struggles and challenges have been numerous; I believe only special peo-ple can endure the challenges I've encountered in my life and emerge triumphant.

I truly believe there is a reason unknown to me that I have been chosen for this tumultuous journey; therefore I will con-tinue to do what I do best, care for others constantly asking the Father Almighty for the grace and the courage to carry on. As I struggle to understand the meaning of my life, could it be I have been living my purpose all along?

I would be remiss not to mention my zest for life. I am a simple, beautiful woman, a smart, strong entrepreneur, and often ask myself, *Why me?* Then, I answer, *Why not me? Why should it be someone else? If it were not me, it would be someone else; would that be any fairer? What's the answer?*

In spite of faith and prayer, I find myself asking forgiveness for my moments of weakness when I question my destiny. Going through this incredible journey—could being a caregiver be the purpose of my life? I believe the Creator knows best and in his wisdom will never give me more than I can bear. No matter what, God gives me the grace and strength to carry on and that's all that matters, so:

My choices

I choose to love myself. I do loving things for myself. I forgive myself for everything. I love myself unconditionally. I feel completely at peace with myself knowing that I've done and given my best and have accomplished a great deal through the grace of God.

Since I am the only person I will have a relationship with all of my life, I choose:

- To love myself the way I am now.

- To acknowledge that I am enough just the way I am.

- To love, honor and cherish myself.

- To be my own best friend.

- To be the person I would like to spend the rest of my life with.

- To always take care of myself so that I can take care of others.

- To always grow, develop and share my love and my life.

Getting help

Now in my senior years the years of stress have taken a toll on my own health. I can no longer do many of the things I once did. In fact, I no longer want to do those things. This is not said to minimize the importance of caring for our loved ones, instead it is a reminder that "no man is an island." I reach out for help. We need help. We need each other.

Perspective

As I look back and reflect upon my life, truly a life of sacrifice and service, I realized that I could only get to this juncture having journeyed through my tumultuous personal experiences. I am forever grateful that the grace of God has sustained and enabled me to endure my many challenges through His divine intervention.

Nothing contributes so much to tranquilize the mind as a steady purpose —a point on which the soul may fix its intellectual eye.
Mary Wollstronecraft Shelley

Acceptance

Working through my struggles I came to realize that acceptance is an important part of happiness. It really defines you, your life and your surroundings. If you want to be happy as I do, you learn to accept the things you cannot change.

Some things we have no control over. The sun will rise and set whether we want it to or not. We learn to accept that reality because we have little or no control over nature. The universe goes on with or without us.

No matter what, life will go on, people will do what they do, everything will continue the way it is, and our only choice is "do I accept it or not?" If we accept it, we go with the flow. We simply let life go on.

If we refuse to accept it, there's usually a struggle within ourselves which results in a feeling of pressure, pain, frustration, anxiety, fear and even resentment. We struggle with ourselves, and the struggle, for the most part, takes place within us where it does the most harm.

When we accept something, it does not mean we like what's happening or are happy about it. It is simply seeing something the way it is and realizing: *That's the way it is; that's what's happening; that's the reality.* It is way easier to accept the things you cannot change. Constantly banging your head against the brick wall only brings endless pain with no resolution

When we do not accept what's happening we invite more pain into our lives and that approach is indeed futile as you will be fighting a losing battle. Non-acceptance allows us to try to be in control of things, to try to control the world. We want to have things our way, but that's not how life works. Sometimes, we cannot even control ourselves, and therefore, cannot hope to control others.

Acceptance is doing what you can, with what you have, with where you are.

Some things we do control. We have control over our own actions, and, to some extent, control over our own thoughts and feelings. I encourage you to focus your energies on those things that you do control. Work to create an environment within yourself that's as loving, peaceful, happy and wonderful as you like in your role as caregiver.

It takes consistent and persistent effort; it is a constant work in progress but never forget that you're creating an environment for yourself and you are definitely worth it, so make it a daily project to preserve your peace and tranquility of mind and body.

As I started to understand how challenging my life as a caregiver would be. I knew in my heart life would never be the same. I am now faced with a new and unusual challenge in the family, multiple sclerosis.

Neither my husband nor myself knew how to tackle this new reality so we continued living life as usual, even though life was anything but! Mum was the word!! Multiple sclerosis was not spoken.

I since learned that when starting off with something new and as challenging as multiple sclerosis, it helps to have support. A good therapist, can be a tremendous help and a healthy place to start. It's beneficial to interact with groups of like minded people whose thoughts are positive; friends and family that stimulate and encourage you.

The most difficult part of my life was a lack of support starting off into the new challenge of multiple sclerosis and my role as caregiver.

I learned that "healing is a matter of time, but it is sometimes also a matter of opportunity." (Hippocrates 460–400 B.C.)

As I grow older and wiser, I learned also that *change* is the only constant in life and it's only our attitude that makes us or breaks us. Ultimately, it's up to you to choose your path.

A positive, mental attitude and a willingness to change circumstances happening in your life, no matter what those circumstances, are truly possible when you change your thought process.

Positive thoughts will bring positive results like health and happiness; caring and sharing; love and kindness; faith, hope and forgiveness; abundance; wealth and prosperity

Negative thoughts will bring you only negative results like, disease; poverty; misery; fear; lack; dislike; alienation; non-communication and indifference.

Negative thinking suppresses the immune system and a weakened immune system invites unwanted dis-ease into your body that makes you sick.

Take an honest look at yourself and your life. It is healthy to do a self evaluation on yourself, on your life and change what is not working. Your decision to invite positive change into your life means you are willing to change old, negative thoughts and habits for positive thoughts and to open up your life to light. Congratulations! Life is change—nothing in life is more permanent than change.

We should be careful to get out of an experience only the wisdom that is in it—and stop there; lest we be like the cat that sits down on a hot stove lid. She will never sit down on a hot stove lid again—and that is well; but also she will never sit down on a cold one any more.

Mark Twain

Coping with caregiver stress

As a caregiver for my husband, I understand stress. Make no mistake, caregiver stress is real, and it has very serious consequences on your health. As a caregiver, you are constantly on the go, and it is easy to put your own health on hold while you continue to provide care for your spouse, mom, dad, family member, relative or friend. Don't let that happen.

While being a family caregiver can be rewarding, it's also very easy to become exhausted and feel completely burnt out. When you begin to feel more and more exhausted each day it is time to listen to your body. Know when you've reached your limit.

When you are stressed out it is difficult to relax and get a good sleep. Your mind wanders, you lay in bed wide awake. As a result, you tend to start the next day exhausted. When you become over stressed, your energy is depleted, and you have difficulty focusing and concentrating.

Stress affects the brain. Because the brain is connected via the network of nerves to every part of the body, your entire body is also affected.

When you are stressed out, the rest of your body feels the impact of your stress. But it also works the other way. If your body feels better, so does your mind and everything about you feels better.

Twelve warning signs

Listed below are 12 warning signs of stress you must not ignore. If you experience any of these warning signs you should seek professional help.

1. You are unable to sleep.

2. You get sick more often.

3. You develop chronic health issues (e.g., high blood pressure, body aches, headaches, upset stomach).

4. You become irritable over little things.

5. You tend to cry over minor upsets.

6. You have difficulty staying calm.

7. You are feeling pressured to carry on.

8. You feel a sense of hopelessness.

9. You lose interest in everything you once loved to do.

10. You are too tired to care, chronic fatigue.

11. You withdraw from socializing.

12. You experience loss of appetite.

Stress affects every organ in the human body. Pay attention to these warning signs now and make adjustments to manage your stress to avoid bigger health issues down the road.

You must take care of yourself first. If you don't, you will be of no use to the person you are trying to care for.

Keep in mind that your stress can be further aggravated if you are working outside the home.

Workplace issues complicating stress

If you work outside the home in addition to your role as a family caregiver, the stress can really multiply.

Work consumes most of our energies. We need to have jobs, so we are not idle, and we can have sense of purpose, and so we can survive in today's world. Work utilizes our talents, supports our family's needs and wants. However, work is also where we tend to be stressed out, with related issues making us weak, and at times, it can even give some of us anxiety panic attacks.

We spend many or most of our waking hours on the job. On the job, you may feel like you're trying to "outrun a roadrunner." On the job, the potential for conflict is high. Most of us encounter difficult people at work; some of us have an "impossible" boss. Competition for the same job can occur. It is there that you first have this mid-life crisis. It is there that temptations abound left and right.

Long hours, looming lay offs, and workplace bullying can cause physical and emotional harm. High job demands, petty office politics, countless hours of overtime, cutbacks in privileges, conflicts with other people, and limited control over your working conditions conspire to raise your stress level. Stress helps no one. For the employee, stress disrupts equilibrium and is the source of any number of emotional, physical, economic and social problems. For the employer, prolonged workplace stress leads to absenteeism, low morale, sickness, dissatisfaction, high employee turn-over, and reduced job efficiency.

The National Institute for Occupational Mental Health cites the following about workplace stress:

- 25% view their jobs as the number one causes of stress in their lives

- Three-fourths of employees believe that workers today have more on-the-job stress than a generation ago

- 26% of workers said they were "felt burned out often" by their job

- Job stress is more strongly associated with health complaints than financial problems.

(Source: "Workplace Issues One Of The Causes Of Stress," http://plrplr.com/78066/workplace-issues-one-of-the-causes-of-stress/ accessed January 23, 2016)

Take care of yourself first

Regardless of where your stress may be coming from, as a family caregiver, you must first take care of yourself. If you fail to do that, you will burn out and ultimately negate your ability to care for your loved one. Your efforts will become counter productive, and you will soon need a caregiver for yourself to take care of you.

If you are experiencing any of the warning signs of stress and burnout, a visit to your family doctor is a wise first step. Your doctor can help you rule out other physical causes for symptoms, provide some guidance on the type of exercise program (see below) that would be appropriate, and provide referrals to other specialists should their services be appropriate.

There are a number of effective ways to combat stress and burn out. One of the most effective—and easiest to overlook or neglect is physical exercise.

Get relief from stress through physical exercise

Physical exercise will improve your overall health thereby allowing you to be of better service to whomever you are caring for. Medical practitioners and health care professionals encourage you to stay physically active.

Regular participation in physical exercise:

- decreases tension and relieves stress.
- improves your physical health.
- helps you better cope with the physical demands of care giving.
- strengthens your immune system.
- improves concentration and overall cognitive function.
- combats fatigue.
- helps you stay alert when you need to be alert.
- helps you sleep when you need to sleep.
- elevates and stabilizes your mood.
- strengthens your self esteem.
- enhances mental health.

Exercise and other physical activity also produce endorphins. Endorphins are chemicals in the brain that act as natural painkillers. They improve your ability to sleep, which in turn reduces stress.

Psychologists studying how exercise relieves anxiety and depression suggest that a 10-minute walk may be just as good as a 45-minute workout. Some studies show that exercise can work quickly to elevate depressed mood in many people. Although the effects may be temporary, they demonstrate that a brisk walk or other simple activity can deliver several hours of relief, similar to taking an aspirin for a headache.

Science has also provided some evidence that physically active people have lower rates of anxiety and depression than sedentary people. Exercise may improve mental health by helping the brain cope better with stress. In one study, researchers found that those who got regular vigorous exercise were 25 percent less likely to develop depression or an anxiety disorder over the next five years. About five minutes of aerobic exercise can begin to stimulate anti-anxiety effects.

Stress and anxiety are a normal part of life, but anxiety disorders, which affect 40 million adults, are the most common psychiatric illnesses in the U.S. The benefits of exercise may well extend beyond stress relief to helping to protect you against anxiety and related disorders.

For more information, see *Exercise for Mood and Anxiety, Proven Strategies for Overcoming Depression and Enhancing Well-Being*, by Michael W. Otto, PhD, and Jasper A.J. Smits, PhD (Oxford University Press, 2011).

Establishing a workout program

The most recent federal guidelines for adults recommend at least 2½ hours of moderate-intensity physical activity (e.g., brisk walking) each week, 1¼ hours of a vigorous-intensity activity (such as jogging or swimming laps), or a combination of the two.

If you have an exercise program already, keep up the good work. If not, here are tips to get you started.

- 5 x 30: Jog, walk, bike, or dance three to five times a week for 30 minutes

- Set small daily goals and aim for daily consistency rather than perfect workouts. It's better to walk every day for 15-20 minutes than to wait until the weekend for a three-hour fitness marathon. Lots of scientific data suggests that frequency is most important.

- Many options for physical exercise are available: yoga, swimming, weight training, treadmill, racquetball, and the list goes on. Find forms of exercises that are fun or enjoyable for you. Extroverted people often like classes and group activities. People who are more introverted often prefer solo pursuits.

- Distract yourself with an iPod or other portable media player to download audio books, podcasts, or music. Many people find it's more fun to exercise while listening to something they enjoy.

- Recruit an "exercise buddy." It's often easier to stick to your exercise routine when you have to stay committed to a friend, partner, or colleague.

- Be patient when you start a new exercise program. Most sedentary people require about four to eight weeks to feel coordinated and sufficiently in shape so that exercise feels easier.

Other stress management suggestions

Remember, if you are experiencing symptoms of stress and burnout, a visit to your family doctor is a good place to start.

You will want to rule out other causes, and discuss any exercise plans.

Don't reach for a chocolate bar for comfort or grab a burger to cope with stress. Instead, try these simple, yet effective techniques to prevent or relieve stress:

- Take care of yourself first. If you don't, you will not be able to care for others.

- Take control of your life.

- Balance your life. Create time for all of your roles, not just your role as a caregiver. Be sure to schedule time just for yourself.

- Take time away from the daily routine to gain a new perspective. This rejuvenates and energizes the body making it possible for you to cope better in your role as caregiver. You will be able to add more value to both yourself and the person receiving care from you.

- Get in touch with nature by walking, biking, hiking. Sit on the bank of the river and listen to the water. Go on nature walks through the parks and nature preserves; enjoy the peace, tranquility and the beauty of everything around.

- Take in deep gulps of fresh air breathing in and out. Breathing in and out as deeply as you can revitalizes and relaxes your mind and body.

- Rest and relax; let your mind go blank—not thinking of anything or anyone.

- Take time out to do things you enjoy. Take time to relax; take in a good movie, go to the spa, read motivational books, do something nice for yourself. Go for a sauna, enjoy a day at the spa (get a facial, manicure, pedicure, and have your hair done), get a full body massage. Look good and feel good.

- Plan properly. Be sure to leave margin in your schedule for unexpected interruptions and delays.

- Surround yourself with friends you can lean on when you need to.

- Work to maintain a positive outlook. Turn to your faith or whatever source of strength you have in your life. No matter what life throws at you, take time to love yourself and keep smiling, meditate, sit and relax with your feet up, think nice thoughts of yourself and of others. When you think good thoughts and do good things, you feel good about yourself, and you make other people happy in the process.

Never forget to love yourself. Whatever it takes to make you happy—take action; make it happen.

Yes, as my swift days near their goal,
Tis all that I implore:
In life and death a chainless soul,
With courage to endure.
Emily Bronte

Caregiver depression

In today's society, there's a greater need for caregivers than ever before—whether it be caring for a spouse, aging parents, children, a disabled family member, a quadriplegic, a neighbor, and so on. Caregivers are taxed to a maximum, and one of the most silent health crises is caregiver depression.

A conservative estimate reports that 20 percent of family caregivers suffer from depression, twice the rate of the general population. It also estimates that former caregivers may not escape the tentacles of this condition after care giving ends.

A recent study found that 41 percent of former caregivers of a spouse with Alzheimer's disease or another form of dementia experienced mild to severe depression up to three years after their spouse had died. In general, women caregivers experience depression at a higher rate than men.

(Source: Family Caregiver Alliance/National Center on Caregiving, caregiver.org)

Care giving does not cause depression, and not everyone who provides care will experience the negative feelings that go with depression. However, in an effort to provide the best possible care for a family member or friend, caregivers often sacrifice their own physical and emotional well being. The emotional and physical demands of providing care can strain even the most capable person. Caregivers can experience a kaleidoscope of emotions including anger, anxiety, sadness, isolation, exhaustion, and guilt. This emotional stress can exact a heavy toll on caregivers.

Caregiver depression should not be minimized

Unfortunately, feelings of depression are often seen as a sign of weakness rather than a sign that something is out of balance. Often times we may hear comments such as "snap out of it" or "it's all in your head." Such comments are not helpful. They reflect a belief that mental health concerns are not real. Ignoring or denying your feelings will not make them go away. Mental health issues are equally as important as physical and emotional health issues and should not be undervalued.

Symptoms of depression

People experience depression in different ways; the type and degree of symptoms vary by individual and can change over time. The following symptoms, if experienced for more than two consecutive weeks, may indicate depression:

- A change in eating habits resulting in unwanted weight gain or loss.

- A change in sleep patterns—too much sleep or not enough.

- Feeling tired all the time.

- A loss of interest in people and/or activities that once brought you pleasure.

- Becoming easily agitated or angered.

- Feeling that nothing you do is good enough.

- Thoughts of death or suicide, or attempting suicide.

- Ongoing physical symptoms that do not respond to treatment, such as headaches, digestive disorders and chronic pain.

Treating depression

Early attention to symptoms of depression may help to prevent the development of a more serious depression over time.

The National Institute of Mental Health offers the following recommendations:

- Set realistic goals in light of the depression and assume a reasonable amount of responsibility.

- Break large tasks into small ones, set some priorities, and do what you can as you can.

- Try to be with other people and to confide in someone; it is usually better than being alone and secretive.

- Participate in activities that may make you feel better, such as mild exercise, going to a movie or ball game, or attending a religious, social or community event.

- Expect your mood to improve gradually, not immediately. Feeling better takes time.

- It is advisable to postpone important decisions until the depression has lifted. Before deciding to make a significant transition—change jobs, get married or divorced - discuss it with others who know you well and have a more objective view of your situation.

- People rarely "snap out of" a depression. But they can feel a little better day by day.

- Remember, positive thinking will replace the negative thinking that is part of the depression. The negative thinking will be reduced as your depression responds to treatment.

- Let your family and friends help you.

The most frequent treatment for depressive symptoms that have progressed beyond the mild stage is antidepressant medication such as Prozac or Zoloft, which provides relatively quick symptom relief, in conjunction with ongoing psychotherapy, which offers new strategies for a more satisfying life. A mental health professional such as a psychologist or psychiatrist can assess your condition and arrive at the treatment most appropriate for you.

(Source: caregiver.org/depression-and-caregiving, Family Caregiver Alliance)

Preventing depression

Respite care relief, positive feedback from others, positive self talk, and recreational activities are helpful in avoiding depression. Look for classes and support groups available through caregiver support organizations to help you learn or practice effective problem-solving and coping strategies needed for care giving. For your health and the health of those around you, take some time to care for yourself.

The return from your work must be the satisfaction which that work brings you and the world's need of that work.

With this, life is heaven, or as near heaven as you can get.

Without this – with work which you despise, which bores you, and which the world does not need—this life is hell.

William Edward Burghardt Du Bois

How to avoid caregiver burnout

The stress care giving creates can quickly turn to burn out if you don't create a plan to avoid burnout.

Self care

Caregivers must always be aware that they can only continue to help their loved ones by first loving themselves. To love yourself is to pay attention to your body's needs. A natural part of living and thriving is to provide essential nutrients, rest and relaxation to your body. When you fail to pay attention to your own health and well being your body will eventually break down. When that happens no one benefits. Instead of you being able to care for your loved one you now need a caregiver to take care of you.

Take care of your own health. Get good nutrition, plenty of sleep, and regular exercise to stay in top health. Wash your hands regularly to prevent colds and flu. Manage your stress with laughter, a prayer or even a deep breath. Nourish your soul with a taste of activities that recharge your batteries such as writing in your journal or gardening. Finally, talk to your doctor if you feel depressed or anxious.

The best strategies to avoid caregiver burnout include preparation, acts of self-care, and reaching out for help. This begins with the courage to start talking openly about care giving so you do not neglect your own health while caring for your loved ones.

A word about beauty

As a caregiver, it is essential that you take care of yourself. Beauty goes hand in hand with self care. For your own self esteem and emotional health, take time to be beautiful both on the inside and the outside. When you look your best on the outside, you feel good on the inside. The result is beneficial to your entire body.

Attention to beauty need not take a great deal of time and effort. Here are a few simple tips to maintain your inner and outer beauty:

- Get enough sleep—at least 8 hours per night.
- Drink plenty of pure water each day—about one ounce for every pound you weigh is ideal.
- Eat healthy balanced meals.
- Exercise regularly—at least three times per week.
- Get enough sunlight, and breathe fresh air.

What is beauty? You are! You are created beautiful. Let your inner beauty shine through!

Community resources

You will want to explore community resources that support care giving. A day program, for example, helps your loved one by providing social connections with peers. Your community may even offer transportation to and from the program. Getting out of the house offers the additional benefit of getting bodies moving. Socializing and exercise are the two most powerful interventions that help your loved ones stay at their best.

Make specific suggestions to friends, family members and neighbors who want to help. You may even want to keep a "help list." When they say, "Let me know what I can do," you have a response:

- "Can you take Mom to her physical therapy appointment this week?"

- "When you're at the store, can you pick up some apples and strawberries?"

- "Can you watch the kids for an hour so I can get to the gym?"

Your well intentioned friends will appreciate specific ideas about how they can help.

Respite care

You should have some plan for respite care. Perhaps another family member or friend can fill in for a few hours or even for a weekend. Hiring a caregiver for respite care may be possible, and, in some cases, long term care insurance or government assistance may be available to help cover the costs.

Respite care is a great and much needed temporary arrangement so you can enjoy a vacation knowing your loved one is safely taken care of.

In some cases, a short term stay at a respite care facility may be an option for your loved one. This elevated level of care may be perfect for the loved one of a family caregiver who wants or needs to get away for a few days or a couple weeks. The last thing a caregiver needs is to be constantly worrying that a mistake was made and the level of care will not be adequate.

To help you make an informed decision on which type of facility better meets your needs check out senior retirement living on the internet. While detailed information is usually available online, you should book an appointment to visit the facility to meet with senior staff members, ask as many questions as you wish, and to clarify any concerns you have.

A good respite care facility should provide three meals daily in a full-service dining room, extensive recreation, housekeeping, laundry, professionally trained nurses and support staff available 24/7, physiotherapy, a house physician, personal care. The facility staff should be prepared to deal with emergencies and other situations that may require medical care outside their facility. These respite services may provide social, cultural, spiritual and educational events, and may offer a wide range of fitness programs. In some facilities, residents can also receive manicures, pedicures, hairdressing and related services. The respite care facility should be audited regularly by the appropriate government agency(ies).

All that is comes from the mind; it is based on the mind, it is fashioned by the mind.

The Pali Canon, 500- 250 B.C.

How to overcome fear & worry

Worry and fear can be a major source of stress for a caregiver. If you are caring for a loved one whose health is unstable and whose future is unpredictable, worry and fear can tug at you throughout the day and keep you awake at night.

In addition, if you are trying to grow as a person, but not achieving the goals you have set for yourself, there may be limiting beliefs that are holding you back. For example, have you ever attempted something new and stopped before you even got started? If so, can you identify the reason? Could it be you were afraid of what others may think of you? Or did you doubt your ability to succeed? These negative beliefs are often rooted in fear or worry.

Someone once defined fear as follows:

> F—false
>
> E—evidence
>
> A—appearing
>
> R—real

When we buy into false beliefs, they become our reality.

Worry is nothing more than a sustained fear caused by indecision or apprehension about the future.

Here are some practical steps to overcome worry and fear.

#1 Clearly define what you are afraid of or worried about. Write in down—put it on paper. The instant you can define your fears clearly by putting them on paper, many of them will simply disappear. Here's why: What was once so big in your mind will look small and insignificant on paper.

#2 Ask yourself: What is the worst possible thing that can happen if this fear or worry becomes true? Make a list. Yes. Write it down on paper beneath your clearly defined worry. Keep writing down everything that comes to mind until you have identified the worst possible outcome.

#3 Once you have completed your list, resolve in your mind that you can accept the worst possible outcome if it comes to that. Accept that worst possibility by telling yourself over and over again: *I can handle it*. This will start to turn things around for you.

Do you realize that 90% of what we worry about never happens? Since 90% of the things we fear will never happen and generally the other 10% will not kill you, understand that you will survive. Think of all the time you spend worrying about stuff that might never happen. This list will help you to clearly see that.

#4 Begin now to make sure that the worst never happens. Put together an action plan of exactly what you need to do to turn things around. By focusing on positive changes and implementing your action plan, your focus will shift away from your fears and toward positive outcomes. You will begin to feel better because now you can do something. Positive action is the only cure for fear and worry.

Try this formula today and see if it will work for you. It has worked for me.

Avoid what is evil, do what is good; purify the mind—
This is the teaching of the Awakened One.
The Pali Canon, 500–250 B.C.

How to use the power of the universe to improve your health

With rising healthcare costs and the increased cost of pharmaceuticals, many caregivers are looking for alternative approaches to staying healthy. One such alternative approach is to apply the Law of Attraction.

The Law of Attraction tells us that what we feel and what we think determine what we experience. Our thoughts become our reality. The Law of Attraction has been discussed on major television talk shows such as *Oprah* and *Larry King Live*.

Using the Law of Attraction, countless people have been able to make big changes in their lives. Watching *The Secret* and learning about the Law of Attraction has helped many people to improve their health. *The Secret* DVD introduced two people who tell their extraordinary story of healing as a result of using the power of the Law of Attraction. (See www.thesecret.tv.)

Here's how it works

Our bodies are made to heal themselves. Determination and will power will help us to use the power of the Law of Attraction and keep us in vibrant health. Of course, that may sound easy, but there is still work involved.

The Law of Attraction teaches that we are vibrational beings, and the universe responds to our vibrations with exact matches

—no exceptions. What we feel and what we think make all the difference. To get well we need to *feel* well. More on this below.

Practical steps

You can take the first steps to help yourself and to improve your health. You can have a healthy body way up into old age.

First, we must believe it is possible. If we think that we cannot change certain health conditions then they probably will not change. On the other hand, if we have a strong will and are convinced that we can get well, this may be possible. There are many cases of persons who have been cured from dreadful deceases without a possible explanation.

Second, you want to do as far as is up to you to live a healthy lifestyle—eat healthy, exercise regularly, get the sleep you need.

Third, educate yourself on the Law of Attraction. Much information is available online, at your local library, at a good bookstore. You may want to check out *The Attractor Factor* by Joe Vitale or *Law of Attraction* by Michael J. Losier.

Fourth, meditate daily for at least ten minutes. This helps you relax your mind and body. It enables you to listen to your inner being and become one with your inner self. It will help you connect things together mentally and emotionally, preparing the way for your healing process.

Fifth, begin changing how you feel and what you think by reprogramming your thoughts. Start saying affirmations that are in harmony with good health and happiness. For example, you might say, "I am a happy person, and I love my healthy and strong body." Say these affirmations daily or throughout the day. Determination to get well will help you along the way.

When saying your affirmations put your feelings and emotions into it! Try to feel how it feels to be strong and healthy. Of course, it may be difficult at first. Feeling healthy when you are not may be challenging. It is, however, a process that will get you to experience a healthier you.

Sixth, supplement these efforts by reading books of success stories of people who overcame severe health conditions. Your body will respond to this and you will see at least an improvement if not total recovery.

It takes time

Using the Law of Attraction to overcome health problems is a wonderful method which has been proven effective for many people. Keep in mind, however, you will probably not experience drastic changes overnight, but if you pay attention to yourself you will notice a difference soon after you start your healing program using the Law of Attraction.

Death is not the greatest loss of life. The greatest loss is what dies inside us while we live.

Norman Cousins

A 10-step guide to create your own anesthesia to numb your pain

It's nearly impossible to carry out your role as a caregiver if you are in chronic pain. Over the years, I've tried many different ways to overcome pain, and by far the best way I've discovered is a combination of hypnosis and mind skills/tools. Let me explain:

Can you remember a time when you had a paper cut and you did not realize that you had it until later on that day when you saw it with your own eyes? It was not until you saw it that it hurt, and you thought, *Ooh, that burns a bit.* This is naturally occurring anesthesia. Your pain was canceled by your mind. The capacity to do this exists within us all.

The technique I use is called the glove anesthesia method, and I share it with you for you to use as you like, when you like.

However, please note this first: You must only use this pain-control technique when you know the cause of the pain. Pain exists to deliver a message. Something is wrong. Figure out what is wrong first, and deal with it if you can. Consult your physician, especially if pain persists.

With that in mind, use this technique to control pain and to remind yourself of how amazing you and your brain really are.

Step #1

Find a comfortable place where you will not be disturbed. Close your eyes, and get yourself relaxed. Focus on your breathing, let your breathing be steady, deep and slow. Imagine relaxing all the muscles in your body one by one and really do take the time required to establish a nice, relaxed, physical state.

Use your imagination, imagine a favorite place, somewhere you feel safe and relaxed. Imagine that you can hear the sounds of that place, see the sights, feel the feelings that you would feel in that place. Use your conscious mind's awareness and focus on each of the muscles in your body; think the word "soften" into each of your muscles. Imagine them melting, softening and allow your mind to be peaceful.

Take a good few minutes to do this; indulge yourself and relax.

Step #2

Develop a strong sense of purpose right now. Using your internal dialogue, remind yourself and tell yourself that you have the power and ability to be in control of any sensations in your body and mind. You really do! Tell yourself that you accept that you are in control of your own mind. Focus on and imagine the unlimited power of your mind, tell yourself that you can send numbing sensations into any part of your body. Develop a sense of belief in yourself and in the power of your own mind. Encourage and empower yourself.

Imagine that these words of personal power and belief that you say to yourself are being delivered to the deepest depths of your mind. Imagine that they've been accepted on every level of your body and mind.

At this stage, also tell yourself that the word "anesthesia" is your key trigger word for a conditioned response later on.

Step #3

Now we begin to invoke the glove anesthesia. Begin by concentrating upon your dominant hand, really focus on it to the exclusion of all else. Notice the tiniest of sensations within it. Begin to imagine that using your attention your dominant hand is free of all feeling. This needs some time and concentration.

You may wish to use your imagination to imagine that your hand is encased in ice. Truly imagine those feelings.

Step #4

Separate your hand, in your mind, from the rest of your physical body. Think of it as detached from your physical being. Continue to focus your attention upon your hand and allow it to lose all feeling.

Using your internal dialogue again, tell yourself that your hand is becoming numb. No feeling at all. Inside your mind instruct your hand to go to sleep. Tell it to go to sleep. Be aware of all the unusual sensations that are in your hand as you focus upon it and keep all your focus and concentration upon it.

Tell yourself that every breath you take seems to cause your hand to become so numb you cannot feel your hand at all. You just can't feel your hand at all because it is numb. No feeling. Your hand is numb. Tell yourself that with authority and belief.

Step #5

Now, you're going to transfer this lack of feeling to the part of your body that you desire to feel numb and have the anesthesia in. So when you are sure that you have created the correct level of numbness in your hand you're going to raise your hand and place it upon the part of your body you want to feel numb.

When you do this, you'll transfer this numbness to that part of your body. So then go ahead and raise your hand and touch the part of your body you want to become cool and numb. Maybe imagine the numbness as a color that you are spreading into that area. Imagine that part of your body being filled with that color and creating that numbness. Imagine all the sensations of numbness are being transferred into that part of your body. Release the numbness into that other part of your body.

Spend some moments doing that properly and thoroughly now. As you do it, give yourself a time limit that this is going to last for. Naturally, you do not want that part of you to be numb forever. So make sure that you set yourself a time limit when your self-induced anesthesia will end.

Step #6

Now that you have transferred the calming, soothing, numbing coolness, and you're physically feeling better and better in that area. Really enjoy the sensations and marvel at your own amazing self. Imagine coolness permeates the area. Imagine you experience wonderful relief in that area. Breathe deeply and relax completely.

You may even repeat a little mantra of support to yourself at this point: "Calm, cool, soothing, numbing sensations permeates the area. Better and better. Numbness. Relief. Numbness." Use words that appeal to you the most.

Step #7

When you have maintained the state and are sure that you feel really good, say the word "anesthesia" to yourself. In this way, each time you use this word in future occasions, when you have the right intention and conditions to do this again, saying the word will bring the resources of this session to make the next time even better. Breathe deeply, embrace the sensations in your body and mind and repeat the word to yourself. Trust that each time you choose to use it in the future, it has a wonderful effect of enhancing and amplifying your control over your anesthesia.

Step #8

And it's time to focus the incredible power of your imagination by imagining yourself doing this even better next time. Imagine that you feel more and more in control of your own mind each time you do this. Experience the joy in this realization. Create every detail of this future occasion in your mind, including your reaction and the reactions of others. And in so doing you communicate your desire to the levels of mind that will assist you in manifesting this natural anesthesia better and better each time you do it. Each time you use that word when practicing your anesthesia, tell yourself it works more and more profoundly and powerfully.

Imagine yourself really feeling good about this and what you can do with the power of your own mind.

Spend a few moments quietly doing this.

Step #9

When you have fully absorbed all you can from this wonderful experience, open your eyes and remember all that has been communicated.

Step #10

Practice, practice, practice! The more you practice, the better and more thorough it is.

You may want to practice doing this on your arm. Prior to doing it, pinch your arm until it hurts to gauge what your pain tolerance level is in that arm. Then when you have it anesthetized, test how different the sensations are.

Neither a lofty degree of intelligence nor imagination nor both together go to the making of genius.

Love, love, love, that is the soul of genius.

Mozart

Making changes

As a caregiver, it's easy to fall into a rut. The demands of your everyday life make it difficult for you to make the changes you need to make for your own health and well being, and, ultimately, for the good of the person you are caring for. I understand this. Yet, I also know that we stop growing when we stop making changes. Life doesn't get better unless and until we are prepared to make the changes we need to make.

So, how do we get off dead center?

Books, courses, seminars, and the like all have their place, but some people become "seminar junkies" who go from guru to guru looking for answers but never seeing change. You don't want that to happen to you.

Start here. Understand that no expert, no book, no course is going to change your life. None.

Only you can change your life. Only you hold that power. The only way your life changes is this: You must decide to change.

Begin by taking responsibility (not necessarily the blame or the credit, but the responsibility) for whatever is going on in your life—the good, the bad and the ugly. However it found its way into your life, it's up to you to figure out what to do with it. You alone have the power to change it.

Decide what you are going to accept in your life, and what you will not accept. Determine what you want and what you don't want. Decide who you want to be. Create a plan. Take the first step—today. Take a step toward your goal every day, even if it's a baby step. You get from here to there by moving, so take a step in the direction you want to be.

Do it. That's the most important step of all. Just do it. That separates achievers from dreamers, success from mediocrity.

Remember that failure is a stepping stone to success. A child doesn't stop learning how to walk because she fell down. She gets back up and tries again. Failure is an event, not an identity. Get back up. Try again. Try a different way. You can do it. You will do it, if—and only if—you decide you will.

The dangers of caregiver denial

When a family members shows signs of dementia or some other chronic condition requiring care, denial is a common response.

Why do we go into denial? We don't feel prepared on multiple levels to deal with the realities of this new situation. It's easier to pretend that the challenging situation doesn't exist.

Although denial is meant to protect us, unfortunately, it does much more harm than good.

Dangers of denial

Accident risk for the patient. If the family member being cared for needs supervision, but that supervision is not provided, falls, cuts, burns, and other accidents could result. If a patient has declined to another level of care, and needs intervention—say a walker, and we don't face that reality, we place that person at risk.

Patients get lost. When not properly supervised due to caregiver denial, family members with memory issues can wander off, get disoriented, get lost, and find themselves in a great deal of danger.

Medication overdoses/underdoses. The person you are caring for may need someone to administer medication. If that family member has Alzheimer's, dementia, or any of several other health challenges, too much or not enough medication could be taken, or medication could be taken at the wrong times, or mixed in a way that is dangerous to the patient.

Medical intervention too little, too late. When we are in denial we tend to minimize the need to get professional help. Symptoms may indicate a need to consult a physician, but that consultation doesn't take place. As a result, the patient can be at risk, and problems that could be easily solved or prevented become major, even life-threatening.

Poor nourishment. Family members who need care may not be able to (or may not remember to) shop for food, prepare meals, and eat healthy if they are not given the appropriate level of care.

Family conflict. When some family members are in denial and others are facing reality, conflict escalates.

Financial trouble. Some patients—especially those with memory issues—cannot be trusted handling their own finances. They forget to pay bills. They become easy targets for people who would take advantage of them financially.

Legal issues. The time to get legal papers—medical power of attorney, wills, living wills and so on—is early on when the patient is able to think through the issues and make an informed decision. Denial can delay these important steps, and create serious challenges for the family later on.

Elder abuse or patient abuse. When caregivers are in denial about the level of care needed by the family member, they may try to bully them into taking on responsibilities (like cooking, cleaning, dressing, etc.) that they simply are not capable of doing.

Missed opportunities for family relationships. Elizabeth Longseth writes, "I was in denial with my father and I avoided visiting him as often as I used to. It was so painful seeing this brilliant geneticist no longer able to hold a long, intelligent conversation. His communication skills became that of a young child. So instead of visiting every month like I had been, I came every other month or every three… Deep in denial, I lost the chance to create special memories with my father."

(Thanks to author Elizabeth Lonseth for much of the content in this chapter. See http://www.aplaceformom.com/blog/9-19-14-dangers-of-denial/, http://www.aplaceformom.com/blog/9-28-15-dangers-of-caregiver-denial/. See also http://dailycaring.com/caregiver-stress-are-you-in-denial/ and http://www.caregiverstress.com/family-communication/solving-family-conflict/denial-a-common-emotion-family-caregivers/.)

Caregiver health challenges and burnout. Refusing to face reality can have serious consequences for your own health as a caregiver. You need to pay attention to your body, and get the help you need in time so that you stay healthy. Caregivers have a significantly higher mortality rate, and much of this, in my opinion, can be traced to denial and a failure to get help when you need it.

Denying that you need help is a major reason for caregiver burnout. A refusal to get the help you need escalates your levels of stress, causes you to start feeling resentment, and creates stress-related health issues for you. Every caregiver needs the help and support of a care-giving team. You are no exception. Extreme fatigue, chronic stress, poor health, depression—these things can be avoided. Get help.

Preventing and dealing with denial

Family meetings and meetings with professionals to understand the needs of the family member receiving care, the options available for that care, and the needs and limitations of family caregivers is a must.

Family members in denial need to understand that doing nothing has consequences. Not to decide is to decide. Fear can sometimes overrule logic, but nobody wants to create a situation that's more challenging for everyone.

It may help to keep a journal so you can get your feelings on paper where you can begin to face what you're feeling and the circumstances you are in. If you think you might be in denial, seek out a friend or loved one—someone you trust—and discuss your feelings with that person.

Get educated. There are many resources that can help you better understand what you're dealing with, the options available, and the support that's out there to help you with your care giving journey.

Denial is NOT the same thing as positive thinking. Having a positive attitude is great, but denying reality is not. If stress is climbing, if you're feeling resentful, if your health is declining, if your world has shrunk down to only you and the family member you are caring for, then it's time to get help.

There are two tragedies in life. One is to lose your heart's desire. The other is to gain it.

George Bernard Shaw

Blessings come from suffering

The life of a family caregiver is not easy. In addition to all of your other responsibilities, a new responsibility has entered your life—the care and well being of a family member. Who plans to spend years—perhaps the rest of your life—caring for an adult family member? Most of us don't. It can feel like an unexpected and overwhelming burden—a 24/7 burden with no reprieve, no clear end date, no break, no escape. It can feel horribly unfair.

Coming to terms with this burden is critical for any caregiver. Unless we learn to cope with what we perceive to be the unfairness of life, we will be miserable. And when the caregiver is miserable, he or she tends to make everyone in the family miserable.

So what's the solution? Do we adopt a Pollyanna-style optimism coupled with a denial of reality? I don't think so.

For me and for countless others, my faith has empowered me to come to terms with my own set of circumstances. These two passages of scripture have helped me gain a different perspective:

Humble yourselves therefore under the mighty hand of God, that in due time he may exalt you. Cast all your anxieties on him, for he cares about you. Be sober, be watchful. Your adversary the devil prowls around like a roaring lion, seeking some one to devour. Resist him, firm in your faith, knowing that the same experience of suffering is required of your brotherhood throughout the world. And after you have suffered a little while, the God of all grace, who has called you to his eternal glory in Christ, will himself restore, establish, and strengthen you.

1 Peter 5:6-10 RSV

Count it all joy, my brethren, when you meet various trials, for you know that the testing of your faith produces steadfastness. And let steadfastness have its full effect, that you may be perfect and complete, lacking in nothing. If any of you lacks wisdom, let him ask God, who gives to all men generously and without reproaching, and it will be given him. But let him ask in faith, with no doubting, for he who doubts is like a wave of the sea that is driven and tossed by the wind.

James 1:2-6 RSV

I've come to believe that unpleasant circumstances are not a punishment, but rather a sacred trust from God. God trusts us enough to believe that we will see our suffering from His perspective.

What does that mean? To begin with, we'll understand that our suffering is temporary, because everything in this life is temporary. It doesn't go on forever. Furthermore, suffering gives us opportunity to grow—if we allow it to. Yes, some people become embittered by their suffering. But others triumph through it. By inviting God into our suffering, we gain patience, perseverance and perspective. We gain empathy and a depth of compassion that we would otherwise never have. We gain a deeper understanding into the human condition and, with it, an ability to connect with others on a more meaningful level.

This doesn't mean that we invite or attract suffering. Of course not! None of us wants to suffer—rather we embrace the life we have been given. We play the hand we've been dealt the best we possibly can. Part of that process is refusing the lies that suffering sometimes wants to tell us—lies like: *You're not worth protecting. You're all alone. Something bad is going to happen to you. Nobody cares.* And so on. We refuse to succumb to hopelessness, and instead ask ourselves, *What opportunity is today—this moment —providing for me? What can God and I do with this set of circumstances?*

If you take this approach, you will emerge triumphant. Over time, you'll find that the things that once troubled you cannot trouble you any more. They lose their ability to make you suffer. People and circumstances that would at one time make you miserable lose the power to do so. You become immune. You gain a kind of inner strength that empowers you to overcome.

I haven't always liked my circumstances. But I can honestly say that I am a better, stronger person today because of them.

One more thought: I see pain and suffering as two very different things. Pain is a physical response to something wrong in the body. As I've indicated elsewhere in this book, there are ways to coping with pain. Suffering is an emotional response to a circumstance we find difficult to accept. That emotional response can also change. For me, the key has been to invite God into my circumstances, and do my best to see those circumstances from His perspective.

Humour is a prelude to faith and Laughter is the beginning to prayer.

Reinhold Niebuhr

How to manage guilt so guilt serves you not imprisons you

Many caregivers feel guilt. Guilt can paralyze you. But it can also propel you.

Guilt is your mind's way of drawing attention to something in your life that needs your focus. Unfortunately, guilt is often not well calibrated, so our guilt stops us instead of motivating us.

Your values create for you an image of the ideal you—the you you want to be. But when the choices you make and the choices the ideal you would make don't align, guilt is the result. You promised to be there for your child's recital. But care giving responsibilities pulled you away at the last minute to a medical appointment. Sure you were placed in a no-win situation, but the result is guilt.

Sometimes the ideal you that you construct in your mind doesn't make room for the legitimate needs the real you experiences. The real you needs to sleep. You need to eat. You need exercise. You need a day off. You need time to yourself and time with friends. You need to laugh, and sometimes you need to cry. You need a safe place to fall apart once in a while. Work out a plan so your needs get met. You will be in a much better place to care for the needs of your loved one if your needs are being met.

You may be angry about your loved one's illness—angry at yourself (*I should have recognized the symptoms earlier and done some-*

thing), angry at God (*This is so unfair!*), angry at your loved one (*Why did you need to get this disease?*). Feeling this anger, processing it constructively, and moving on is all part of the larger process of coming to terms with your role as a caregiver.

Five ways to cope with guilt

Here are five things you can do to manage caregiver guilt so that it serves you rather than imprisons you:

#1. Be honest with yourself. Be honest about the guilt you are feeling as well as any other emotions that are present. Facing what is really there is an important first step. Put your feelings into words. And understand that some things may *feel* true even though you know they aren't *actually* true. It's important to own your feelings—they're part of you, and they need to be looked at honestly.

#2. Give yourself room to be human. Some days you may feel angry. Some days you may feel guilty. Okay. That's not the end of the world. That doesn't mean that you want to export all of your negative feelings on everyone around you, but it does mean that we're all human. We all have bad days. It's okay. Let yourself be you.

#3. Change what you can change. Do your best to identify the cause of your guilt. Do you have needs that aren't being met? Do you need to make a different set of choices that better match your values? Take the action you need to take—meet your needs. Do you need a day off? Find someone to provide that much needed respite care? Do you need to change some of your choices? Think it through, create a plan, make it happen.

#4. Get help. Phone a friend. Reach out to your support network. Do you need to unload? Find someone safe where you can share what you are really feeling. Maybe you need to call a family meeting and discuss how everyone can work together to make sure that everyone's needs are being met.

#5. Review and reconstruct the ideal you. You are a growing person. As you grow, your values grow with you. Maybe the ideal you isn't so ideal. Maybe it's not only unrealistic, but also unhelpful for you to try to provide 24 hour care six or seven days a week. Your values need to work in the real world—the world where you really live. What's truly important to you? What kind of legacy do you want to leave?

You will provide better care for your loved one when you take care of yourself first. Guilt may be part of the journey, but use that guilt to bring you and your family to a better place.

(Thanks to Vicki Rackner MD or "Dr. Vicki" for the concepts in this chapter. http://www.e-mailtherapy.com/caregiver-guilt-counseling.htm)

The mind is its own place, and in itself can make heaven of hell, a hell of heaven.

Milton

The freedom of forgiving others

Resentment and bitterness can kill a caregiver. While caregivers may have many reasons for hurt and anger, these negative emotions, if allowed to fester in our lives, not only rob us of the enjoyment of life, they can actually create life-threatening disease within. Someone likened refusing to forgive others to putting yourself in prison as a way of punishing someone else who hurt you.

Do you see any problem with that?

Here are some thoughts on forgiveness adapted from *Rediscover God* by Dwight Clough. (Reprinted with permission of the author.)

In response to the offenses against us—both real and imagined —we can create a well of bitterness inside. The result is terribly destructive; we intend to nourish, but we pollute instead. Forgiveness empowers us to live and love from a position of abundance. Bitterness robs us of that abundance and forces us to ration out love to others from a position of scarcity. Forgiveness is foundational. Furthermore, we have an obligation to forgive those who wrong us, an obligation that God takes very seriously.

Forgiveness is often characterized as a difficult choice achieved by a heroic struggle of the will. I would like to suggest to you that this is misleading. Forgiveness is not difficult. Forgiveness is impossible.

An example: Some years ago, a friend and I were helping a woman who had been horribly abused to forgive the perpetrator of that abuse. She sat across from us, closed her eyes and concentrated on her words. "I choose to forgive," she said. Clearly she was mustering all her willpower as she forced herself to forgive an offender for his acts of abuse.

She tried to force herself to forgive. This is the way Christianity is commonly practiced. Do what you know is right whether you feel like it or not. But I believe that God wants to do a better work, a deeper work in the lives of His people. I believe that Jesus will show up for His people when they lay aside their own efforts and rely totally on Him.

I sensed that her anger toward this offender was still solidly in place. So I asked her to focus on whatever feelings came up when she thought about this man and his offenses.

Sure enough. Despite her best efforts to forgive, the anger remained as strong as ever.

I said to her, "Look inside your heart, and let me know if there are any reasons why you can't give this anger to Jesus."

She thought about it and said, "If I give my anger to Jesus, I feel like I'm letting the offender off the hook."

With her permission, I brought her objection to Jesus, and invited the Lord to deal with this reason she couldn't release her anger. "What about this?" I asked the Lord. "Will giving her anger to You let this guy off the hook?"

A moment later, she smiled. The reason was gone. She said. "I'm ready to give this anger to Jesus." Soon the anger was gone, and, in it's place, she felt soothing peace and joy. After a few more moments of letting Jesus share with her how much He cared about her, she was delighted to forgive the offender.

She walked away flooded with peace and joy, thanking God for His goodness to her.

What a contrast! On one hand she tried to do what was right and was left with anger, bitterness and a cheap substitute for the real power of God. On the other hand, when Jesus was brought into the broken places in her heart, He made everything new.

Myths about forgiveness

Myth #1: forgiving an offense benefits the offender but taxes the offended.

Truth: Forgiving an offense empowers the offended.

It is to a man's glory to overlook an offense (Proverbs 19:11). Forgiving frees us from the kind of bitterness that saps away our energy and turns our whole world a muddy gray. Yes, forgiving benefits the offender, but only because it forces the offender to deal directly with God. No longer are you and I standing between God and the offender. Now God can deal with that person and use all of His ingenuity to turn that life around.

Myth#2 To forgive you must go into denial about your anger.

Truth: Forgiveness is not about burying your anger.

Yoda's advice to his Jedi followers is almost the worst thing you can do with anger. Many people believe that Christians should bury their anger, deny it, suppress it, "forget" about it. None of those things work. The anger remains and festers inside like a cancer. Eventually it comes back out as illness, depression or an explosion of violent emotion.

Myth #3 Forgiveness minimizes offenses.

Truth: Forgiveness is not about rationalizing or minimizing the offense.

Telling ourselves that "it wasn't really that bad" or "he didn't really mean to..." or "she was under a lot of pressure when she..." does not resolve the anger or result in forgiveness. The offense is what it is. In Matthew 18:23+, the king began by taking account. He measured the debt. He took an honest look at what was really owed.

Myth #4: You forgive by saying "I forgive you."

Truth: The words "I forgive you" do not automatically result in forgiveness.

The words "I forgive you" in themselves are not a magic incantation and do not automatically result in forgiveness. Forgiveness is sometimes thought of as an act of the will, summoning the willpower to say those words aloud. True forgiveness goes much deeper than that. When true forgiveness takes place, the anger isn't buried; it's gone.

Myth #5: Forgiveness invites an abuser back into your life.

Truth: Forgiveness is NOT reconciliation.

Forgiveness is not reconciliation. If someone raped my daughter, I would want her to eventually come to the place of forgiving the offense so she would no longer need to carry the burden of bitterness. But asking her to have a relationship with the rapist would be absurd, unless the rapist himself underwent a dramatic and verifiable transformation.

In fact, someone I care about was raped. Although I think forgiveness is an important part of the healing process, I did everything in my power to protect the victim from having any contact with the perpetrator. I also championed the prosecution of the man who committed the crime. Simply because we may choose to forgive does not mean that the legal system should forgive. No. They have a different responsibility before God. It isn't our job to dispense justice, but it is their job to dispense it. We are not vigilantes; we are citizens.

Myth #6: You can forgive everyone who has ever hurt you in one act of forgiveness.

Truth: Blanket forgiveness doesn't work.

We don't, for example, typically forgive Uncle George in ten minutes when he abused us for ten years. Multiple offenses from a single person require multiple acts of forgiveness. As a rule, we need to visit each place where anger remains and forgive each specific offense.

Myth #7: If forgiving others is therapeutic for you, then something must be wrong.

Truth: Doing the right thing (forgiving others) is also right for you.

Forgiving someone who wrongs you for your own sake is not selfish. Rather it is obedience. Some people reject biblical commands merely because they are therapeutic. Some make the mistake of thinking that God does not want us whole. To not forgive is to harbor bitterness that will hurt many. This has nothing to do with justifying the actions of a perpetrator. On the contrary, when we truly forgive, we have the emotional strength to do what is appropriate in regards to the perpetrator —as in the rape example I provided earlier.

How do we forgive?

We find the anger, feel it, connect it to the offense and ask ourselves the question: Is there any reason that would keep me from giving this anger to Jesus. If there is, bring those reasons to Jesus and let Him deal with them. When He does, then the reasons will be gone. When all the reasons are gone, then you can release the anger for that offense to Jesus. Once the anger is gone, forgiving that offense—canceling the debt—is easy.

One should sympathize with the joy, the beauty, the color of life—the less said about life's sores the better.

Oscar Wilde

Positive thinking and a new direction

In the early morning hours of February 4, 2015, I got out of bed unable to sleep. I was at a low point in my life—feeling overwhelmed, exhausted, angry and sad. It was scary. I simply could not carry on much longer on my present path of darkness. I felt the need to do something meaningful for myself. In addition to being a caregiver, I needed mental stimulation. I was at my wit's end, and I needed to make a positive change immediately.

I got on the internet, looking for a new direction in life. I was attracted to home based businesses for several reasons. First, a home based business fit my lifestyle as a caregiver. Second, I figured the right company would provide the support of positive people with similar goals and values. Third, the right business would provide much-appreciated added income.

As I researched home based businesses, I stumbled upon Wealthy Affiliate. Determined to change the course of my life I signed up for one month's free trial. Within a week I became a premium member. Since joining WA, I have enriched and transformed my life. I am energized and empowered as I enter a new chapter of life. I have incredible mentors from whom I learn, and I love interacting with the people in this vibrant, online community. In turn, I am sharing my experience as a caregiver on the world, wide, web, paying it forward. Here's the website I use to do that: http://caringforcaregiver.com. Browse through if you so desire. Your comments will be gratefully acknowledged.

The outcome? I have come to truly appreciate the value of adversity and challenges in my life. Could it be that these challenges are the catalyst for bringing out the best in us?

I wake up each morning gratefully knowing I am in a beautiful place today, and I am making the best of it. I have life and the ability to make a difference in our world. I will not focus on what I lack. Instead, I will be thankful for all the blessings and good things I already have. Today, I am focusing on creating new value.

With an open heart and mind and a huge smile on my face I open my life to all good possibilities without any restrictions or conditions.

Moving along with the life I have, I channel my energies into enjoying the simple, beautiful things in life. This is my life and I delight in who I am.

Here's the link to how I got started on this incredible adventure: http://www.wealthyaffiliate.com?a_aid=3f15dc22

Look on the bright side

The important thing here, of course, is not that you join Wealthy Affiliate or any other home business—instead that you find ways to see the positive, that you always look on the bright side.

Remember: Positive thoughts create positive energy, empowering you to better face and overcome the roadblocks and challenges life throws our way. You can turn your lemons into lemonade. No matter what situation presents always look to find a positive outcome.

Every painful experience can be a learning opportunity. These experiences make you stronger, wiser, smarter and better able to handle the next challenge life throws your way.

Is this concept simple? Yes. But don't mistake simple for trivial. Once you truly "get" this and make it part of your life, it changes everything.

Successful people understand that they alone control their attitude. They don't give other people the power to make them feel angry, bitter, upset or anything else. This gives them the freedom to pursue their goals without being weighted down with all this excess emotional baggage. The beautiful thing about understanding is this: It doesn't cost anything. You are totally free to do the same.

You too can incorporate positive examples into your life and change your outcomes. Think positive thoughts, do positive acts of kindness, focus on good memories of the past and on realistic future plans that you can look forward to with passion and pleasure.

In spite of illness, in spite even of the archenemy sorrow, one can remain alive long past the usual date of disintegration if one is unafraid of change, insatiable in intellectual curiosity, interested in big things, and happy in small ways.

Edith Wharton

Your identity

With all the challenges that care giving presents, you need a strong psychological and spiritual anchor to rise above these challenges, to function, and—some days—just to keep your sanity.

I find that anchor in my faith, and in a strong sense of my own identity. Knowing who I am helps me to put the daily struggles that go with being a caregiver into perspective. A clear sense of your own identity will help you preserve your equanimity as you wrestle with the stresses of your role as a family caregiver.

There are many ways to look at identity, but I like this short piece entitled "What I believe about you" from the book by the same title by Dwight Clough. (Reprinted with permission of the author.)

You are no accident.

You have been in God's heart and in His plan

from eternity past.

God is at work in you.

All the broken places in our lives are simply opportunities

for God to show His great love and transforming power.

God never fails.

He is smarter than our enemy,

stronger than our addictions.

God likes you.

He likes hanging out with you.

You are deeply treasured.

No one can take your place in God's heart.

God will satisfy all your desires with good things.

The signature of God is on you;

you are His creation,

and God doesn't make junk.

You were created to live forever,

designed to make a difference,

engineered for excellence.

God is with you.

You have what it takes.

You are here for a purpose.

You carry Jesus into our broken world.

You are the answer to someone's prayer.

You are the friend someone longs for.

You are the difference your world needs.

When you took the hand of Jesus,

you entered into life.

You became indestructible,

undefeatable,

incorruptible.

All the powers of hell

might line up to take you down,

but Jesus pushes those bullies up against the lockers,

and you walk by unharmed.

You are a royal son, a regal daughter of God.

And thank you for being my friend.

We must cultivate our garden.

Voltaire

Do you really know what you want to be in life?

Being a caregiver doesn't mean that you give up your own hopes, dreams and goals. Not at all! You may need to make accommodations for your role as a caregiver, but that role is not a dead end street that prevents you from going where you want to go in life.

But here's the problem: Most people don't know what they really want in life.

Can you make a list—in order of importance—of the ten most important things you want to do, to have or to be in life?

Understand the value of such a list. When opportunities come knocking at your door, this list helps you decide which ones to pursue. Your top-ten list will help you set goals and make plans. It will answer the question, "What am I going to do for the rest of my life?"

Knowing what you want helps you get what you need. For example, sometimes people with a chronic or life threatening disease get well by pursuing their dreams. Their dreams give them a reason to live and to live well. By knowing what you want and pursuing it, if your health is lost, it may "mysteriously" return.

How to create your top-ten list

Start by brainstorming. Write down everything you want to do, everything you want to have, everything you want to be. Don't edit at this point. Don't toss anything out. Include everything. Remember to list material, emotional, mental, physical, relational and spiritual goals. You may want to take several days to make your list complete.

Once your list is complete, it's time to begin pruning. How many things do you truly want? Did you write down any items just because you thought you *should* want them? "Should want" and "want" are two different things.

Did you include anything that might really be a symbol for a deeper want or need? For example, if you want an expensive car or home, why do you want it? Do you want it to meet an unconscious emotional need? If so, can you identify that need and find an even better way to meet it?

What are your priorities? Remember, you can have anything you want; you just can't have everything you want. If you aim for everything, you hit nothing. That's why we need to narrow the list. Ask yourself: Am I willing to do the work required to achieve this goal? Am I willing to make a plan and carry it out? Is this in line with who I am and why I'm here? If the answer is no, then cross it off.

Check your list to see if two or more items are in conflict with one another. Gaining a slim, trim, healthy body, for example, may be in conflict with "eating all the dessert I want to eat every day." And there may not be enough hours in the day to become both a professional football player and a concert violinist at the same time.

Rate the items on your list. Which items receive an "A"? (I want this very, very much.) Which items receive a "B"? (I want this a lot.) And so on.

How many "A's" do you have? If you have more than ten, you can eliminate all the "B's" and "C's." Otherwise, keep eliminating less important items until only the top ten remain.

Out of the ten that remain, choose the most important. Copy it to a fresh list—your final top ten—as your #1 most important goal. Do the same with each of the remaining nine, until you have a top ten list ranked in order of priority.

After each goal on your top ten list, answer one important question: How will I know when I've reached my goal?

Be specific so you'll know when to cross it off your list to make room for another.

Well done! With your completed top ten list, you've create a life plan.

It is the chiefest point of happiness that a man is willing to be what he is.

Desiderius Erasmus, 1465-1536

Setting goals

Once you have your top ten list (see previous chapter), you'll want to set and achieve goals to get what you want in life.

Keep in mind, you will only achieve your goals if:

(1) You know precisely what you want. Vague dreams do not get accomplished. Achievable goals do.

(2) You are passionate about your goal. You will face many obstacles and setbacks; you need the passion to persevere.

(3) You have a realistic plan for achieving your goal. Success does not magically appear. You must take certain steps in the real world for it to happen.

Here are five realities you need to embrace to achieve your goals.

1. Be clear and precise about what you want. What will achieving your goal look like? Be as specific as possible. During World War II, a prisoner spent a great deal of time imagining what his life would look like as a resident of Los Angeles. Every day, he imagined that potential reality. One day, the front gate of his prison camp happened to be open for a few moments. He walked out, escaped to freedom, and moved to Los Angeles to live his dream.

Be specific about your desired outcome. "Your success will be a measure of your clarity, since an achievable goal plan cannot be created around a nebulous dream," writes Dr Jill Ammon-Wexler in "5 Steps to Goal Setting Success" (http://www.4hb.com/20050104053909.html).

Be specific about things like income, net worth, lifestyle, finished product, or whatever your dream entails. A clear mental picture will give you the focus you need to achieve your goal.

2. Make the necessary sacrifices. There are only 24 hours in a day. If you're going to make changes, you'll need to subtract before you can add. You'll need to take things out of your schedule before you can add things to your schedule. Keep in mind that everybody (including you) needs sleep, recreational time, relationship time, family time, as well as making a living time. You also need to account for the time you spend in your care giving role. But there are 168 hours in a week, and achieving a new goal means shuffling a few things around.

3. Refocus on your goal daily. Your brain is accustomed to the status quo. Changing your outer reality means you must first change your inner reality. That's why you need to come back to your goal every day. You'll need to override the mental images and subconscious messages that keep you locked in the way things are if you're going to break free into the way you want things to be. Recommit to your goal daily. Stand your ground. Insist on what you want. Don't back down.

4. Build passion. Passion is like fuel for the engine of success. Passion gives you the power to climb the mountain of achievement. There are all kinds of obstacles—both internal and external—between you and what you want. Passion gives you what you need to go over them, go around them, go under them, or just knock them down. Passion helps burn new neural pathways in your brain to construct that new reality for you.

5. Every day take a small step toward your goal. Without action, your goal remains in your imagination. Specific steps get you from here to there. The steps are mostly small, but they are all necessary. If you want to walk from New York to Los Angeles, you can do it, but it will require about six million steps. People have done it, and you can achieve your goal as well—you just gotta take that first step, then the second, and so on. Remember, we don't take all the steps at once. We just take one at a time. Take a step today.

Don't let fear or worry hold you back. Face those fears. Identify the negative beliefs that drives them. Tell yourself the truth.

What is fear?

F-false

E-evidence

A-appearing

R-real

Don't buy into false beliefs. Instead, identify those negative beliefs. Clearly define what you are afraid of or worried about. Write down what *feels* true, even though you know it isn't true.

Many times, fears and worries dissolve simply by naming them and putting them on paper. What seemed so big in the corner of your mind now seems weak and insignificant.

For those fears that remain, ask yourself: What is the worst that can happen?

Again, write it down. Make a list. Identify those worst possible outcomes. Most of what we worry about never happens. This list helps bring that reality into focus.

You can handle it. Almost certainly the worst that could happen falls within the category of things you can handle if you need to. It might be unpleasant, but you can handle it.

That isn't to say you should accept it. No! Make a plan right now to make sure that the worst that could happen doesn't happen.

Overcome your fears, and achieve your goals!

How many cares one loses when one decides not to be something but to be someone.

Coco Gabrielle Chanel

Visualization

Your ability to visualize what you want greatly enhances your chances of achieving your goals. Visualization techniques have been successfully used to achieve all kinds of goals—from winning Olympic gold medals to feeling more confident when speaking in front of a group of people. You can use mental imagery to become happier, stronger and more effective.

Visualization is a powerful tool for attracting what you want, but few people know how to use it.

Here are some techniques that will help you visualize:

1. Specify what you want. As humans, we are always imagining, constantly conjuring up images in your mind. For many people, those images are negative, or, at best, neutral. They may be focused around bills we may be struggling to pay, or people we wish we could impress. However, a far more powerful use of your imagination is to visualize your success—imagine what you want. Be specific.

2. Practice in your mind. Our brain experiences well-crafted images much the same way it experiences reality. Maybe this is why professional golfer Jack Nicklaus practiced each shot in his mind before taking it. In fact, According to Alejandro Reyes, "Australian Psychologist Alan Richardson made a little experiment. He took a group of basketball players, divided them in 3 groups and tested each player's ability to make free throws. The first group would practice 20 minutes every day. The second would only visualize themselves making free throws, but no real practice was allowed. The third one would not practice or visualize. The results were astounding. There was significant improvement on the group that only visualized; they were almost as good as they guys who actually practiced." ("Does Visualization Really Work? Here's Evidence That It Does," http://expertenough.com/1898/visualization-works)

3. Imagine each step. A 2011 study by scientists at McGill University, in Montreal, found that when told to eat more fruit, people who envisioned every step of the process (reaching for it, biting into it, enjoying it) were more successful than those who only generally thought about eating more fruit. Imagining each step may create neural pathways so the action feels familiar when you actually carry it out.

There is no failure except in no longer trying.

Elbert Hubbard

Successful action

As we've seen in previous chapters, you must take steps—action—in the real world if you are going to achieve your goals.

Remember: How much you want something is defined by your actions. If, for example, someone says to you that he wants health, you look to see what he is doing about it. Is he actively involved in his own healing? Is he doing everything he can to promote healthy ideas, healthy thoughts, feelings and healthy actions in his life? Is he exploring more and more options for greater health? If he is, he really does want good health. If he isn't, then, maybe he doesn't really want what he says he wants.

To think or feel that you want something does not necessarily mean that's what you want. What you really want is that which you actively manifest in your life, what you make real through action.

If you think you want something *and* you're not really doing much to get it, you have three choices:

1. You can go on the way you are: pretending you really want what you think you want. I don't recommend this because it causes frustration, hurt and anger. (*Why me? I never get what I want.*)

2. Give up the goal. You recognize that your time is spent seeking other things, therefore, you must want them more than you

103

want this, so for the time being—let this one go. This is a perfectly acceptable option, if you're content with it.

3. Do whatever is necessary to reach your goal. As you work towards the goal, certain mental, emotional and physical objections will be raised. No matter what complaints your mind, emotions and body bring forth, if you know you need to do it, do it anyway. Gently, lovingly—but firmly teach the objecting parts of you that you have a new goal, a new priority, and that your actions will now be in alignment with achieving that goal.

When taking action, understand the difference between being efficient and being effective:

- Efficiency gets the job done right.
- Effectiveness gets the right job done.

It doesn't help to take a shortcut if you're headed in the wrong direction. Once you determine what you want, make a plan and put it into motion. Do what you need to do. Start and persist.

Here are eleven principles of action that will help you:

1. Divide each goal into achievable steps. If you want to write a book, you need to decide on reader, do some research, write an outline, write the first chapter, and so on. The next achievable step might be to talk to a few people to see if there is interest in the topic you want to write about.

2. Put these steps on your calendar. Whether you use a calendar app, or write things down in an appointment book, your goals stay in your head until you take some kind of action.

That means figuring out a time to do what you want to do—not all of it at once, but a piece of it—a first step.

3. Be flexible. Nothing ever goes exactly according to plan. Know that up front. And it really is okay. You grow, you change, your goals and your project grows and changes with you.

4. Be willing. What you are *willing* to do you will become *able* to do.

5. Don't allow your emotions to stop you. Your emotions are important because they signal something happening inside just like a "check engine" light tells us to look under the hood. But don't let your feelings paralyze you. Anxiety or inner resistance is a common barrier we all must break through in order to grow. We all are resistant to change at some level, but without change there is no growth, and without growth, we won't achieve our goals.

6. Turn fear into fun. Excitement and fear are cut from the same cloth. They belong to the same emotional continuum. Use fear to your own advantage. For example, professional speakers welcome nervousness before they go on stage because it gives them added energy to connect with an audience. When you feel "fear," call it "excitement" instead. Instead of saying, "I'm afraid," say "I'm excited." Consider "fear" your ally. Consider it preparation energy. Let it keep your mind focused, your energy up, and your attention clear. It may be just what you need to help you do new and exciting things.

7. Turn won't into will. Stubbornness and determination are two sides of the same coin. Peter McWilliams (see note below) writes, "Both include steadfastness, constancy, power and drive. It's a matter of turning "won't power" (stubbornness) into "will power" (determination.) When you find yourself being stubborn (I don't want this), find out what you do want and, using the same energy move toward it. *Will* past your won't. *Do* past your don't."

8. Model it. Pretend you are teaching your plan to someone else. Set the example. Do what you do with excellence. In reality, you are teaching. McWilliams writes, "You are teaching various parts of your mind, body and your emotions to live more fully."

9. Find stepping stones. In life's highway, all of us experience unexpected detours. Don't think of these things as roadblocks. Instead, consider them opportunities. You get to take the scenic route! You get to learn something new. You get to grow and become stronger. Welcome challenges, and let them mold you into a better person.

10. Ask. Ask for what you want. Do you need help? Ask! Do you need someone to show you the way? Ask! Other people don't know what you need until you ask them. No one can read your mind, but many are willing to help—if you ask.

11. Be gentle. Be gentle with yourself and with others. Do not be so obsessed with your goal that the process is miserable for you and everyone around you. Do what you do with love. Remember the African proverb: You go faster alone, but farther together. Let others around you feel the warmth of your love. That way, when you arrive at your destination, you will have friends there to greet you.

If health, happiness, joy and/or love is on your list of goals, focus only on what's good, what's right, what's pleasant and what's worth appreciating around (and within) you. By doing this, you will be doing a great deal to promote health, happiness, joy and love.

(Many of the thoughts in this book, particularly in this chapter originated from an excellent book that I highly recommend by Peter McWilliams: *You Can't Afford the Luxury of a Negative Thought: A book for people with any life-threatening illness-including life*, Prelude Press, 1988.)

The destiny of mankind is not decided by material computation. We learn that we are spirits, not animals, and that something is going on in space and time, and beyond space and time, which whether we like it or not, spells duty.

Winston Churchill

Commitment

The ability to make and keep promises is what will move you from the life you have today to the life you want tomorrow.

In previous generations, important agreements could be sealed with a handshake because most people would never think of violating their word. Today, billions are spent on contracts and contract disputes, and many times people end up in court because someone failed to keep their promise.

Someone said, "If you want to be happy in life, you keep all your commitments and don't expect other people to keep any of theirs." (http://goo.gl/0YXPCe)

Our integrity is measured in part by how well we keep our promises. When we don't keep our word trust erodes—not only do others begin not to trust us, we begin to distrust ourselves. We don't believe in our ability to keep our own promises. Our confidence is replaced with self doubt.

There are three main reasons why people break agreements or commitments. First, they should have said "no" when they said "yes." This often happens because they fear the disapproval of the other person. But the problem is this: by getting someone else's temporary approval, they lose their own self approval. Second, sometimes it's just easier not to put in the work to keep the commitment. But this always backfires. The little bit of comfort we gain by, say, going off the diet and indulging in unhealthy foods comes back to bite us later, making it twice as hard to get what we want. Third, some people feel a sense of rebellion. They just don't want to be hemmed in by an agreement with someone else, particularly if that person appears to be an authority figure. But rebelling also backfires. Ultimately, it hurts us more than the person we're trying to hurt.

If we've failed to keep our promises (even the ones we make only to ourselves) in the past, we must rectify that by making a new commitment to be a person of our word in the future. We must only make commitments that matter to us, and never make promises we can't keep. Far better to say "no" up front, rather than promise and fail to deliver.

If you do make a commitment, write it down. It helps you to remember your promise, and keeps you clear on exactly what you did promise. Putting it on your calendar also helps to avoid scheduling conflicts.

If something gets in the way of you being able to keep your promise, it's so important that you communicate with all parties as early as possible. This gives everyone an opportunity to adjust their plans and to work together toward a common solution.

Bring closure by declaring things finished. Some books you may never finish reading. Some projects you may never complete. If they aren't important, if they're sucking energy and life from you that should go elsewhere, simply declare these things finished and walk away from them. You'll be surprised how much energy you free up for the things that really matter.

Finally, forgive yourself. If you've broken promises to yourself in the past, forgive yourself. Today is a new day. Now is a new start. You are a new you. Let the past go; start fresh. If you've made commitments to others and haven't kept them, make it right if you can. If you can't, forgive yourself and move on. This will free up energy to empower you to keep your commitments in the future.

Also, forgive others. People make commitments. People break commitments. It happens. It's never pleasant, but let it go. Expecting others to always keep their promises is (a) unrealistic, and (b) and invitation to irritation. The energy you use up feeling angry and resentful toward that other person could be far better used to move you closer to your own goals.

It is not good enough to have a good mind. The main thing is to use it well.

Rene Descartes, 1637

The winner's walk

When you meet someone new, your perception of the person and what you feel about them is based 93% on body language. A big portion of that body language is seen in how you walk. When you walk like a winner, people feel your presence and know you have something to offer. We all know people who are filled with confidence. They walk like they have just won a gold medal in the Olympics. They walk like they own the street they're walking on. They walk with confidence.

When you walk like a winner, people want to be around you. They feed off your energy. Ask yourself, *Do I present myself as a winner?*

Here are a few secrets on how to walk like a winner:

Walk with your shoulders back, chest out and at a slightly faster pace than usual. This is the key.

Even when life hits you on the blind side (and it does), walk like a winner because your physiology will empower you to move through whatever is mentally frustrating you.

When you walk into a meeting to market yourself or your product, people will feel your confidence and will want to hear what you have to say because they will feel your energy and enthusiasm.

As you continue to master your body language, you will notice an increase in your personal production, making it easier for you to achieve whatever you set your mind to achieving.

I wish to personally challenge you to walk like a winner this entire week and see how things around you change.

Resources for caregivers

Books

The 36-Hour Day: A Family Guide to Caring for People Who Have Alzheimer Disease, Related Dementias, and Memory Loss, fifth edition by Nancy L. Mace, M.A., and Peter V. Rabins, M.D., M.P.H. Originally published in 1981, The 36-Hour Day was the first book of its kind. Thirty years later, with dozens of other books on the market, it remains the definitive guide for people caring for someone with dementia. "Both a guide and a legend."—Chicago Tribune. "Excellent guidance and clear information of a kind that the family needs."—New York Times

ABA/AARP Checklist for Family Caregivers: A Guide to Making it Manageable by Sally Balch Hurme (2015) can help organize the responsibilities that caregivers face. In one place, you'll be able to record and update the myriad details you need to keep track of. And if you don't know where to start, this invaluable tool tells you, step by step, what you need and why. You can easily personalize the to-do lists, either in the book or electronically, and have them available for quick reference for your care giving team—family, friends, aides, and medical, financial, and legal professionals.

Alzheimer's Disease and Other Dementias by Nataly Rubinstein. Alzheimer's disease can be crippling for a caregiver. Exhausting emotional and financial resources, it often creates a diagnosis of despair. Nataly Rubinstein offers hope.

Alzheimer's: The Identity Thief of the 21st Century by Robert B. Schaefer. This is a true, inspiring story of love directed toward anyone—family or professional who is affected by this horrendous disease. It is filled with faith, hope, humor, understanding, survival and realistic suggestions as experienced by the average person and their care-partner following a diagnosis of dementia and/or Alzheimer's.

The Best Care Possible: A Physician's Quest to Transform Care Through The End Of Life by Ira Byoch, MD puts a human face on a national crisis: the way in which our healthcare system makes illness and dying far more difficult than they ought to be. Dr. Byock introduces readers to patients whose lives are threatened and the doctors and caregivers who are singlehandedly shaping how families experience loss. The book puts a human face on the real, heart-wrenching realities of being seriously ill in the United States. The message is at once sobering as well as hopeful and consistently life-affirming.

The Caregiver's Companion: Caring for Your Loved One Medically, Financially and Emotionally While Caring for Yourself by Carolyn A. Brent MBA walks readers through the crucial issues of moving their aging loved ones into an assisted-living facility as well as discussing emotional, medical, legal, and financial issues with them. Checklists are provided for gathering important information. A particularly helpful chapter delves into the frequent dilemma of dealing with the loved one's resistance to even talking about these issues." (Library Journal review)

Caregiver's Handbook by DK Publishing is a compassionate and comprehensive resource for anyone who needs to take care of an elderly person at home. This reference offers constructive, illustrated guidance for first time and beginning caregivers, including information on essential first aid, advice on selecting professional help when needed, and dealing with a variety of common conditions.

The Caregiver's Handbook by Sallie Voyles is a tutorial, with worksheets, for those finding themselves thrust into the position of primary caregiver. Authored by a professional strategic planner, this workbook helps identify priorities and create a plan to better control a very emotional situation. Content includes the development of a plan to handle appointments, documentation, identification of resources, the creation of a support system, legal considerations and estate planning. The hospital section provides recommendations for being the advocate for your loved one and communicating effectively.

The Caregiver's Path To Compassionate Decision Making: Making Choices For Those Who Can't by Viki Kind, MA. This award winning book provides information and strategies to use to empower you to make the difficult decisions. The book's decision-making process gives caregivers confidence, courage and peace of mind.

The Caregiver's Toolbox: Checklists, Forms, Resources, Mobile Apps, and Straight Talk to Help You Provide Compassionate Care by Carolyn P. Hartley and Peter Wong (2015) is your guide to cool apps and online tools, insider tips on how to reduce your medical bills, your privacy rights as a caregiver, where to go for free and low-cost help, and much more. It clearly shows which tools will relieve your stress, and those that may add stress. Available here: http://goo.gl/kOiPDs. See also the authors' website here: www.caregivers-toolbox.com.

A Caregivers Guide to Lewy Body Dementia by Helen Buell Whitworth, MS, BSN, James A. Whitworth is written in everyday language, and is the ideal resource for caregivers, family members, and friends of individuals seeking to understand Lewy Body Dementia.

The Caregiving Trap: Solutions for Life's Unexpected Changes by Pamela D. Wilson draws on the author's life and professional experience supporting thousands of overwhelmed and frustrated older adults and family caregivers. The book provides a realistic view of care and the complexities of the healthcare system. Wilson offers levity and sensitivity while addressing issues few want to talk about—aging, care giving, and death.

Come Back Early Today: A Memoir of Love, Alzheimer's and Joy by Marie Marley, PhD. This colorful, award-winning memoir offers hope and illustrates practical solutions to 14 problems Alzheimer's caregivers typically face—everything from denial, diagnosis, and difficult behaviors to nursing home and hospice care. See also www.comebackearlytoday.com.

Dare to Care: Caring for our elders by Cheryl Carmichael. An easy-to-read reference for family caregivers—helps keep your loved ones living in their own home as they age. Learn about Supervisory, Personal, Memory Loss and Palliative types of care. Six additional chapters cover fundamentals of care giving.

The Dave Test: The Raw Look At Real Faith In Hard Times by Fredrick W. Schmidt. When life is at its tattered edges and you are faced with seemingly impossible decisions, this is a set of searingly honest questions you ask to become the best, most honest self for you, friends and family. Instead of resorting to stained-glass language or offering false hope, take The Dave Test.

A Deeper Perspective on Alzheimer's and other Dementias: Practical Tools with Spiritual Insights by Megan Carnarius RN provides a unique insight into patient needs as well as numerous helpful suggestions for the caregiver as they experience the various stages of dementia diseases and the physical, emotional and spiritual demands. Carnarius is a noted memory care consultant whose expertise is regularly sought out in the designing and managing of care facilities and as a family consultant.

The Delicate Balance: A Mindful Approach for Professional and Family Caregivers by Phyllis Quinlan offers guidance to heighten awareness of the dangers of caring too much.

Dementia: The Journey Ahead: A Practical Guide for In-Home Caregivers by Susan Kiser Scarff. Within a year of receiving her husband's diagnosis, Susan Kiser Scarff had a classic case of caregiver burnout. She couldn't concentrate at work. Friends drifted away. Overwhelmed, she struggled to make the transition from Red's wife to his protector, nurse, and mother. Susan's experience as a first-time caregiver, recorded in these pages with grace, wisdom, and humor, prove just how much there is to learn: finances have to be handled a different way in case the patient decides to make a lone trip to the bank; aggressive behavior is a constant threat; safety becomes a concern in every aspect of daily living

Diary of a Mad Caregiver by Rebecca Grace Collins articulates what many caregivers think, but are afraid to express. Gain a new perspective on the "madness" of care giving. Turn your stressed emotions into joy and worship. Make this book your own personal diary where space is provided for your thoughts.

The Emotional Journey of the Alzheimer's Family by Robert B. Santulli, MD, and Kesstan Blandin, PhD. Incorporating over thirty years of experience with Alzheimer's patients and their families with current medical knowledge, the authors chart the complex emotional journey of the Alzheimer's family from the onset of the disease through the death of the loved one. They discuss the anger that rises in the face of discordant views of the disease, the defenses that emerge when family members are unwilling to accept a dementia diagnosis, and the common emotions of anxiety, guilt, anger, and shame.

The Fearless Caregiver: How to Get the Best Care for Your Loved One and Still Have a Life of Your Own by Gary Barg is a practical, sympathetic and comprehensive guide published by the experts at Today's Caregiver magazine shows caregivers how to be an informed, effective, and fearless caregiver while still having time for yourself.

The Fifth Season: A Daughter-in-Law's Memoir of Caregiving by Lisa Ohlen Harris describes the author's experience caring for her mother-in-law with COPD while raising four young children.

Final Journeys: A Practical Guide for Bringing Care and Comfort at the End of Life by Maggie Callanan is the guide we all need to understanding the special needs of the dying and those who care for them. From supporting a husband or wife faced with the loss of a spouse to helping a dying mother prepare her children to carry on without her, Callanan's poignant stories illustrate new ways to meet the physical, emotional, and spiritual challenges of this difficult and precious time. She brings welcome clarity to medical and ethical concerns, explaining what to expect at every stage. Designed to be your companion, resource, and advocate from diagnosis through the final hours, this book will help you keep the lines of communication open, get the help you need, and create the peaceful end we all hope for.

God Signs: Health, Hope and Miracles, My Journey to Recovery by Suzy Farbman. When the author appeared on Oprah as an expert on relationships, she was at the height of success as an author. Yet, doctors revealed that her body was failing. Facing life's worst fears, Suzy called her colorful circle of friends and charted a personal course toward healing. Suzy found great doctors and spiritual awakenings. She discovered God reaching out to her in Godsigns on a daily basis. This warm, suspenseful and often funny memoir has a universal message: We can find hope if we open our eyes to Godsigns all around us.

Guide for Caregivers by Benjamin Pratt. These are short, easy-to-read sections packed with wisdom and practical help! This book is designed to let readers jump in almost anywhere and explore at their own pace. Considering the millions of people worldwide who are caregivers, this book also is great for small-group study.

Help Wanted: Caregiver: A Guide to Helping Your Loved One Cope With Serious Illness by Laura Pinchot provides a guide to help those who have been tasked with caring for a loved one, friend, or family member. This book offers a primer on in-home care as well as options for institutional care, the next logical step as the scope of care becomes too much to handle. You will also find information on financial and legal issues as well as the challenges caregivers face in their relationship for the person in their care.

I Know How Hard You Work: A Journey Through Stroke Recovery by Paul Sybert relates the author's inspiring journey from a debilitating stroke to his remarkable return to health, while helping other stroke survivors learn to cope.

Inside Assisted Living: The Search for Home by J. Kevin Eckert et al. draws on interviews with residents, family members, staff, and administrators to illuminate day-to-day life in different types of assisted living residences.

Joy-Spirations for Caregivers: Dialogues with God of Hope and Encouragement by Annetta Dellinger, Karen Boerger, George L. Richardson gives hope as you read honest feelings from a caregiver's heart, feel the depth of God's love from His responses, and reflect on stories of encouragement for the challenges and frustrations of care giving. It's a treasure chest for the caregiver.

Leaning Into Sharp Points: Practical Guidance and Nurturing Support for Caregivers by Stan Golberg, PhD is a comprehensive guide filled with real-world wisdom for every stage of caring—from diagnosis, treatment, and decline to mourning and recovery.

Lessons for the Living: Stories of Forgiveness, Gratitude, and Courage at the End of Life by Stan Goldberg. A hospice volunteer shares the amazing things he learned from those approaching the end of life.

Lessons From The Ancients: A Humorously Helpful Guide For Caregiving by J Dyess Calhoun. Make your care giving easier and more enjoyable. A quick read, this family caregiver shares how-to lists resources, humor, inspiring stories. Support and classes for caregivers by phone, web.

Life in the Electric Chair: A Man And His Wife Explore A Life On Wheels by Dan West. I used to do a lot. Now, I have no balance and I've been in wheelchair over 8 years now. Life has changed, but I manage to live well.

My Complete Caregiving Organizer: Tools for Managing the Challenges of Caregiving by Pat Dranchak puts the information you need for taking control of care giving at your fingertips. Create a personal health record, develop a care plan, manage services, coordinate your care team, and handle emergencies. With simple forms and step-by-step instructions. Available in print or digital format. Winner 2011 Caregiver Friendly Award, Today's Caregiver Magazine.

My Doctor Book: A Personal Medical Records Organizer by Mary E. Carlton is an important resource to assist in the prevention of medical errors. This organizer is for anyone who is a caregiver, has a chronic condition, is about to undergo a surgical or medical procedure, or is monitoring routine preventive care. The book will alleviate caregiver stress and empower you to participate in treatment decisions, empowering you to protect yourself, your loved ones and those in your care.

No Saints Around Here: A Caregiver's Days by Susan Allen Toth. Wrenching, at times darkly funny, and always deeply felt, Toth's intimate account of her husband's final eighteen months with Parkinson's reflects the realities of seeing a loved one out of life—all intricately interlocking parts of the act of loving and caring for someone who is fading away. No Saints Around

Here is the beginning of a conversation in which so many of us may someday find our voices.

Nursing Homes and Assisted Living: The Family's Guide to Making Decisions and Getting Good Care second edition by Peter S. Silin. The author approaches his subject with compassion and sensitivity, guiding family members through the process of finding the best possible care. "Practical and valuable information at a difficult time."—Arizona Daily Star

OK Now What: A Caregiver's Guide to What Matters by Sue Collins, R. N. & Nancy Taylor Robson provides life planning resources for family caregivers. See oknowwhat.net.

The Silverado Story: A Memory-Care Culture Where Love is Greater than Fear by Loren Shook, Stephen Winner. Life doesn't have to end when Alzheimer's dementia or other memory-eroding diseases take hold. At least that's what Alzheimer's futurists Loren Shook and Steve Winner believed. But it wasn't until these two men, from widely divergent backgrounds and living three thousand miles apart, came together that their ideas were put into action and their theories were put to the test—with stunning results. They brought living back to people stricken with memory impairing ailments, and loving back to families who thought they had lost a precious part of themselves.

To Love What Is: A Marriage Transformed by Alix Kates Shulman. After her husband suffers a life-altering brain injury, Alix Kates Shulman must learn to care for him without losing herself. Despite ongoing anxieties and setbacks, she reorganizes their world and priorities to enable them both to lead surprisingly fulfilling lives, as recounted in this memoir of crisis, love, and hope.

The Tough & Tender Caregiver: A Handbook for the Well Spouse 1st Edition by David Travland Ph.D., Rhonda Travland. Private, Powerful and Practical solutions minimizing guilt to reclaim joy without abandoning responsibilities.

Transform Your Loss: Your Guide to Strength and Hope by Ligia M. Houben. A self-help book that deals with difficult life transitions or losses and provide a mind-body-spirit guide of eleven principles on how to transform it. It can be used by layperson or professionals. Also available in Spanish

Warriors, Workers, Whiners, and Weasels: The 4 Personality Types in Business and How to Manage Them to Your Advantage by Tim O'Leary is a must read for every entrepreneur, business owner, manager, and worker wishing to learn more about themselves, take advantage of their best traits, and protect themselves from those who could sabotage their career. O'Leary uses a mix of light-hearted humor with a fiercely intense attitude to combine a business book and a self-help book in an exciting fashion.

When Caring Takes Courage: An Interactive, Compassionate Guide for Alzheimer's and Dementia Caregivers by Mara Botonis

When My Mother No Longer Knew My Name: A Son's Course in Rational Caregiving by Stephen L. Goldstein is packed with down-to-earth practical advice and tips to make care giving manageable-even joyful. There's even a unique self-assessment guide so caregivers and potential caregivers can benchmark and enhance their ability to manage the often lonely, challenging, unpredictable, and overwhelming roles they may assume.

When The Time Comes: Families with Aging Parents Share Their Struggles and Solutions by Paula Span. This compassionate, inspiring guide will enable you to care for your parents with joy, and help them age with dignity and grace.

Who Cares? A Companion Guidebook For The Family Caregiver's Journey by Elizabeth Rawson, M.A. Tired, frustrated as a caregiver? Learn the truth: it's OK to take care of you! A fantastic new guide book of helpful ways to THRIVE with inspiring support and renewal.

You Can Do It: A Stroke's Survivor Guide to Independent Living by Daniel A. Holst. For the caregiver and stroke survivor, it covers stroke causes, associated emotional effects, and rehabilitation. A significant portion is devoted to the many activities that Dan learned to do with one-hand.

You Want Me To Do What? Journaling for Caregivers by B. Lynn Goodwin. Are you a caregiver experiencing stress? B. Lynn Goodwin's book gives encouragement, easy instructions, and over 200 sentence starts to help you process and explore. Become a better caregiver. Experience the relief and hope that journaling brings.

Your Wife Has Cancer...Now What? by Carson Boss covers effective support techniques, dealing with difficult emotions, intimidating household chores and step by step financial guidance and more. Six husbands share their stories. The book will give you a quick blue print of what to expect so you can customize your own plan of action in becoming and effective caregiver for your wife, yourself and family.

See also "Today's Caregiver Book List" at

http://www.caregiver.com/bookclub/index.htm

Book descriptions taken from Amazon, from CareGiver.com and elsewhere online.

Websites

Information gathered from each website or otherwise online

AARP Home & Family Caregiving page

http://www.aarp.org/home-family/caregiving/

My Top Tips for Caregivers, as Seen on 'Today' Show

http://blog.aarp.org/2015/11/05/amy-goyer-advice-for-care-givers/

12 Resources Every Caregiver Should Know About

http://www.aarp.org/home-family/caregiving/info-08-2012/important-resources-for-caregivers.html

Handy list of support, services and tips for caregivers

AARP Online Community: Discuss issues with other caregivers in the online community.

Caregiving Tools

http://www.aarp.org/home-family/caregiving/caregiving-tools/

AARP Caregiving App: Share, scan, save and schedule all of your loved one's health needs – all in one handy app. Available on iOS, Android and web.

Caregiving Resources

Caregiving Question and Answer Tool

Caregiving Locator Tool: Search for home health, assisted living, nursing home, hospice and adult day care options near you.

Long Term Care Cost Calculator: Calculate costs for long-term care by area or by type and length of stay.

Caregiving Resource Center - State-by-State Guide

State-by-State Advance Directives

CRC Caregiving Glossary Tool: Terms you should know when caring for a loved one.

Pill Identifier: Unsure what your pill is? Enter its color and shape information, and this tool helps you identify it.

Affordable Care Act-Tool: Health Law Answers: Use this personalized tool to learn how the Affordable Care Act can benefit you and your family.

Medicare Q&A: Get fast access to the Medicare answers you're looking for.

Social Security Benefits Calculator

Benefits QuickLINK: Find programs that help save money on health care, medication, food, utilities, children's health costs and more.

Family & Caregiving Webinars

Make Your House a Home—for Life: Find information and tips on how to keep your home in top form for comfort, safety and livability.

AARP Driver Safety

Alzheimer's and Dementia Caregiver Center

http://www.alz.org/care/

Their store

http://shop.alz.org/Learn-and-Play/Books-and-Games

Local groups & resources:

http://www.alz.org/apps/findus.asp

Alzheimer's Association

www.alz.org

800-272-3900

Information and support for people with Alzheimer's disease and their caregivers. Operates a 24/7 helpline and care navigator tools.

Alzheimers.gov

www.alzheimers.gov

The government's free information resource about Alzheimer's disease and related dementias.

ARCH Respite Network

www.archrespite.org

Find programs and services that allow caregivers to get a break from caring for a loved one.

Caregiver Action Network

http://caregiveraction.org/

Resources from the Caregiver Action Network, including a Peer Forum, a Story Sharing platform, the Family Caregiver Tool Box and more. CAN also provides support for rare disease caregivers at http://www.rarecaregivers.org

Other Key Resources

Resources for Caregivers-2007 Edition (PDF)

Aging Parents & Common Sense – 5th Edition (PDF)

Aging Parents & Common Sense Resource Directory (PDF)

Supports for Single Parent Caregivers Literature Review (PDF)

Caring Today, Planning for Tomorrow (PDF)

Planning for Your Retirement and Long-Term Care (PDF)

http://caregiveraction.org/about-can

The Caregiver Action Network is the nation's leading family caregiver organization working to improve the quality of life for the than 90 million Americans who care for loved ones with chronic conditions, disabilities, disease, or the frailties of old age. CAN serves a broad spectrum of family caregivers ranging from the parents of children with special needs, to the families and friends of wounded soldiers; from a young couple dealing with a diagnosis of MS, to adult children caring for parents with Alzheimer's disease. CAN (formerly the National Family Caregivers Association) is a non-profit organization providing education, peer support, and resources to family caregivers across the country free of charge.

Site includes a discussion board:

http://caregiveraction.org/forum

Topics include:

Dealing With Caregiver Depression—Up to 50% of caregivers experience symptoms of Depression. How do you handle it?

Dealing with Medical Professionals—Getting doctors to pay attention to us can be difficult. What techniques have worked for you?

I'm a New Caregiver…What Do I Do?

Life After Caregiving

Technical and Practical Advice for Caregivers

Working Through Your Frustration and Isolation—Frustration and isolation are often considered two of the biggest personal issues for family caregivers to deal with. What helps you get past these difficult emotions?

Caregiver Resource Network

http://www.caregiverresource.net/

From the website:

The Caregiver Resource Network is a collaboration of 150 West Michigan organizations dedicated to providing for the needs and welfare of family and professional caregivers within the community. The Caregiver Resource Network is facilitated by the Grand Rapids Community College Older Learner Center and Area Agency on Aging of Western Michigan, which administer Title IIIE Older Americans Act National Family Caregiver Support Program.

CareGivingAnswers

http://www.caregivinganswers.com/

Ask any question- it's free

Caring.com

www.caring.com

Caring.com is the leading online destination for family caregivers seeking information and support as they care for aging parents, spouses, and other loved ones. Caring.com offers helpful content, advice from leading experts, a supportive community of caregivers, and a comprehensive directory of eldercare services. Caring.com's carefully researched and expert-reviewed content includes advice from a team of more than 50 trusted leaders in geriatric medicine, law, finance, housing, and other key areas of healthcare and eldercare.

Caring.com's Steps & Stages offers a free guide to Alzheimer's care. Expert advice and practical tips provided in a Custom Care Guide and e-newsletter help family caregivers learn what to expect, what to do, and how to cope with Alzheimer's.

Caring.com also publishes findings from research with family caregivers at http://www.caring.com/about/news.

Financial Steps for Caregivers

WISER (Women's Institute for a Secure Retirement)

Financial Steps for Caregivers: What You Need to Know About Money and Retirement is designed to help you identify financial decisions you may face as a caregiver. The decision to become a caregiver can affect both your short-term and long-term financial security, including your own retirement. For more information on planning for a secure retirement, please visit http://www.wiserwomen.org.

Eldercare Locator

www.eldercare.gov

800-677-1116

Connects caregivers to local services and resources for older adults and adults with disabilities across the United States.

http://www.eldercare.gov/Eldercare.NET/Public/Index.aspx

Are you a family caregiver in need of information or assistance? Are you interested in learning more about the programs and services that may be of assistance to you or your loved one? The Eldercare Locator, a public service of the U.S. Administration on Aging, is the first step to finding resources for older adults in any U.S. community. Just one phone call or Website visit provides an instant connection to resources that enable older persons to live independently in their communities. The service links those who need assistance with state and local area agencies on aging and community-based organizations that serve older adults and their caregivers.

Family Caregiver Alliance

https://www.caregiver.org/

An information rich site for caregivers. Their publications

https://www.tfaforms.com/394066

Reports on care giving state by state across USA

https://www.caregiver.org/caregiving-across-states-50-state-profiles-2014

Programs and Services Overview

https://www.caregiver.org/programs-and-services-overview

From the website:

FCA's work intersects three key areas: caregiver services, policy and research. But across all agency programs, the services and products developed and delivered are based on real needs of real caregivers—those families we hear from and work with every day. Specific business lines include:

Caregiver Services on the regional and national levels include: Bay Area Caregiver Resource Center: FCA works most closely with family caregivers in the San Francisco Bay Area counties of: San Francisco, San Mateo, Santa Clara, Alameda, Contra Costa and Marin. We offer comphrensive consultation services that result in an action plan for families with ongoing follow up from clinically trained staff. Understanding current and future needs of the family and the relative needing care, coupled with expert information and interventions that improve family functioning are hallmarks of FCA service delivery. Often home visits are arranged that combine an assessment of family needs and the home environment for possible modification to cover safety and ease of care concerns. For those families who need more assistance or who are long-distance caregivers, services can be provided through a new fee-based model provided by FCA.

In addition, based on meeting eligibility requirements, family caregivers in the San Francisco Bay Area may be provided with short-term respite and counseling, legal consultation with a qualified elder law attorney as well as high quality education programs that build direct care skills, teach stress-reduction and wellness techniques and provide wide range of up to date topics needed by caregivers. We select from our extensive catalogue of consumer fact sheets, articles and checklists as well as from our regional community services database to prepare a plan that is tailored to the needs of individual families. Our Connections e-newsletter combines the latest news in research, treatment, policy and a round-up of educational opportunities for family caregivers.

For families who live outside the San Francisco Bay Area region, we offer the Family Care Navigator, the first-of-its-kind, comprehensive, online guide to help families locate caregiver support programs and services in all 50 states. Caregivers and professionals find the Navigator an invaluable tool to locate information and specific services in an easy-to-read chart format. And all family caregivers can use our extensive library of fact sheets, articles and checklists and well as participate in our numerous webinars and videos on care giving issues catalogued on our site. Service staff also talk to family caregivers from across the country on our 800 number to quickly assess their needs and tailor the right information and service referral that meets their need.

Policy and Research Activities on the state and national level include: National Center on Caregiving (NCC): FCA's Policy and Research activities include tracking emerging policy trends and legislation at the state and federal levels through our expanded 50 State Profiles. The National Center on Caregiving also engages in research on policy and program areas that recently have focused on the integration of family caregivers in health and social service systems. In the past two years (2012-13), four publications related to various aspects of identification and assessment of family caregivers were disseminated. The NCC continually updates our facts-at-a-glance Selected Caregiver Characteristics that reflect the latest findings in survey and program research. Policy makers, media, program adminstrators, health providers and families can keep current with our Caregiver Policy Digest e-newsletter and our webinars on key policy topics. Technical assistance is available to policy makers and program administrators on system and program development.

FCA engages in advocacy for policies and programs of direct benefit to family caregivers. Working across broad coalitions, FCA has been involved in the passage of noteworthy bills such as the statewide system of Caregiver Resource Centers and Paid Family Leave in California as well as advocated for changes in rules governing assessment of family caregivers for Medicaid waiver programs. Agency staff are represented on key state (CA) and national coalitions, advisory and workgroups that work on a diverse set of issues: quality measures in home and community based services, universal assessment in Medicaid waiver programs, elder justice, Olmstead compliance, workforce development and numerous other topics. FCA is often asked to participate on expert panels relating to care giving topics for use in policy formulation, product development and system improvements in the private and public sectors.

FCA programs are funded by corporate and foundation grants, contracts with government agencies, corporate partnerships and licensing agreements, fees for service and private donations. You can make a donation right now so FCA can help families in need and to continue our work to improve the quality of life for family caregivers and their loved ones where ever they live.

http://caregiver.org/node/3831

Established in 2001 as a program of Family Caregiver Alliance, the National Center on Caregiving (NCC) works to advance the development of high-quality, cost-effective policies and programs for caregivers in every state in the country. Uniting research, public policy and services, the NCC serves as a central source of information on care giving and long-term care issues for policy makers, service providers, media, funders and family caregivers throughout the country.

Family Caregiver University

http://www.caregiverresource.net/uploads/files/Family%20Caregiver%20University%202015%20Class%20Schedule.pdf

Lotsa Helping Hands

www.lotsahelpinghands.com

From the website:

Lotsa Helping Hands is a free care giving coordination web service that provides a private, group calendar where tasks for which a caregiver needs assistance can be posted. Family and friends may visit the site and sign up online for a task. The website generates a summary report showing who has volunteered for which tasks and which tasks remain unassigned. The site tracks each task and notification and reminder emails are sent to the appropriate parties.

Medicare

www.medicare.gov/caregivers

800-Medicare

Provides information about the parts of Medicare, what's new and how to find Medicare plans, facilities or providers.

Medicare caregiver resources

https://www.medicare.gov/campaigns/caregiver/caregiver.html

What every caregiver needs to know [PDF, 155KB]

What does Medicare cover? [PDF, 180KB]

Caring for someone with a chronic illness [PDF, 165KB]

Planning for the future [PDF, 168KB]

What caregiver support is available in my area? [PDF, 206KB]

Taking care of yourself [PDF, 166KB]

Caregiver resource kit

https://www.medicare.gov/campaigns/caregiver/caregiver-resource-kit.html

This section of the Ask Medicare toolkit offers informational resources that can be printed directly from this Web site and provided to caregivers. The resources are designed to help caregivers address challenging issues and work effectively with Medicare to ensure their family members and friends receive the best possible care.

Practical information for caregivers

These materials highlight the basics of caregiving and understanding Medicare.

Ask Medicare brochure: Care for others [PDF, 246KB]

A brief overview of Ask Medicare.

What every caregiver needs to know [PDF, 155KB]

Short facts on caregiving and some of the many resources offered by Ask Medicare.

Ask Medicare: What type of care is best for your loved one? [PDF, 158KB]

A list of terms describing the various types of care for disabled, aged and seriously ill individuals.

Ask Medicare: Billing terms caregivers should know [PDF, 159KB]

Descriptions of common billing and financial terms related to the Medicare program.

Ask Medicare: Questions and answers about Medicare for caregivers [PDF, 151KB]

Information about the Medicare program and other issues that are especially important to caregivers.

Personal caregiver stories

Read stories about caregivers and their approaches for addressing challenging issues.

Tips sheets

These materials will help caregivers manage challenging issues, like paying for care, managing a transition from a hospital to home care setting, managing the stress that can come from caregiving and more.

Ask Medicare: Moving to a nursing home or assisted living facility [PDF, 178KB]

Facts and insights about long-term care options.

Ask Medicare: Planning a transition from hospital to home [PDF, 165KB]

A checklist to help caregivers prepare home environments for individuals who are being discharged from hospitals or other types of inpatient facilities.

What does Medicare cover? [PDF, 180KB]

Basic and essential information about how Medicare works.

Ask Medicare: Is additional financial support available? [PDF, 170KB]

Information for caregivers of family members and friends who are struggling to pay for health care and related costs.

What caregiver support is available in my area? [PDF, 206KB]

Information about local resources and financial benefits that are available to Caregivers.

Taking care of yourself [PDF, 166KB]

Tips to help caregivers address their own physical and emotional needs.

Planning for the future [PDF, 168KB]

Tips on preparing for long-term health, financial and legal issues.

Caring for someone with a chronic illness [PDF, 165KB]

Tips on caring for a loved one with a chronic illness.

Medline Plus—list of resources for caregivers

https://www.nlm.nih.gov/medlineplus/caregivers.html

Links on the website include:

Caregiver Health and Wellness (American Academy of Family Physicians)

Caregiver Stress (Department of Health and Human Services, Office on Women's Health)

Caregivers and Exercise -- Take Time for Yourself From the National Institutes of Health (National Institute on Aging) - PDF

Caregivers and Serious Illness (Administration for Community Living) - PDF

Caring for the Caregiver From the National Institutes of Health (National Cancer Institute)

Coping Checklist for Caregivers (American Cancer Society)

new Coping with Caregiving: Take Care of Yourself While Caring for Others From the National Institutes of Health (National Institutes of Health)

Finding More Help (Long Distance Care-Giving) From the National Institutes of Health (National Institute on Aging)

Help for the Caregiver From the National Institutes of Health (National Cancer Institute)

Respite Care (Administration on Aging)

Taking Care of You: Self-Care for Family Caregivers (Family Caregiver Alliance)

What Is Caregiver Burnout? Easy-to-Read (American Heart Association) - PDF

Adult Day Care (Administration on Aging)

Alternatives to Nursing Homes (Centers for Medicare & Medicaid Services)

Busy Parents and Caregivers Must Care for Themselves (American Heart Association)

Caregiving Video (Centers for Medicare & Medicaid Services)

Caregiving and Sibling Relationships: Challenges and Opportunities (Family Caregiver Alliance)

Caring for Siblings of Kids With Special Needs (Nemours Foundation)

Face the Facts (Administration on Aging)

Guidelines for Better Communication with Brain Impaired Adults (Family Caregiver Alliance)

Hands-On Skills for Caregivers (Family Caregiver Alliance)

Hot Weather Tips (Family Caregiver Alliance)

How to Assemble a Caregiving Team (Fisher Center for Alzheimer's Research Foundation)

Improving Doctor/Caregiver Communication (Caregiver Action Network) - PDF

Information Caregivers Can Use on: Speaking with a Friend or Family Member's Doctor During an Office Visit (Centers for Medicare & Medicaid Services) - PDF

Information for Caregivers (American Health Information Management Association)

LGBT Caregiver Concerns (Alzheimer's Association) - PDF

LGBT Caregiving: Frequently Asked Questions (Family Caregiver Alliance)

Long-Distance Caregiving -- A Family Affair From the National Institutes of Health (National Institute on Aging)

Long-Distance Caregiving -- Getting Started From the National Institutes of Health (National Institute on Aging)

Making Choices about Everyday Care (for Families) (Family Caregiver Alliance)

Managing Care for Adults with Long-Term Medical Illness (Agency for Healthcare Research and Quality)

Medicare and Caregivers: Illness and Hospitilization NIHSeniorHealth (National Institute on Aging)

Medicare and Caregivers: Planning for Medical Care NIHSeniorHealth (National Institute on Aging)

Roles for the Family Caregiver From the National Institutes of Health (National Cancer Institute)

So Far Away: Twenty Questions for Long-Distance Caregivers From the National Institutes of Health (National Institute on Aging)

Support for Long-Distance Caregivers From the National Institutes of Health (National Institute on Aging)

What Are the Caregiver's Rights? Easy-to-Read (American Heart Association) - PDF

What If I Don't Want to Be the Caregiver? (American Cancer Society)

Caring for the Elderly: Dealing with Resistance (Mayo Foundation for Medical Education and Research)

Dental Care Every Day: A Caregiver's Guide From the National Institutes of Health (National Institute of Dental and Craniofacial Research)

Dying Process--A Guide for Family Caregivers (National Hospice and Palliative Care Organization) - PDF

Families with Special Needs: Caregiving Tips (Centers for Disease Control and Prevention)

Family Caregivers and Transportation: A Few Survival Tips (Healthy Living Tips) (Administration for Community Living) - PDF

Family Caregivers in Cancer (PDQ) From the National Institutes of Health (National Cancer Institute)

Guide for Caregivers (National Multiple Sclerosis Society) - PDF

Hospital Discharge Planning: A Guide for Families and Caregivers (Family Caregiver Alliance)

MDA ALS Caregiver's Guide (Muscular Dystrophy Association)

Caregiving Statistics (Caregiver Action Network)

Selected Caregiver Statistics (Family Caregiver Alliance)

ClinicalTrials.gov: Caregivers From the National Institutes of Health (National Institutes of Health)

References and abstracts from MEDLINE/PubMed (National Library of Medicine)

Article: The Littlest Caregivers. Helping Children To Cope With A Parent's...

Article: Celebrations honour caregivers' work.

Article: 'Health is where the home is'.

AAAs (Area Agencies on Aging) & Title VI Aging Programs (National Association of Area Agencies on Aging)

Administration on Aging

Caregiver Action Network

Family Care Navigator: State-by-State Help for Family Caregivers (Family Caregiver Alliance)

National Institute on Aging From the National Institutes of Health

Legal Issues for LGBT Caregivers (Family Caregiver Alliance)

Managing Someone Else's Money: Help for Agents under a Power of Attorney (Consumer Financial Protection Bureau) - PDF

Medicare and Caregivers: Understanding Medicare Billing NIHSeniorHealth (National Institute on Aging)

Medicare Basics: A Guide for Families and Friends of People with Medicare (Centers for Medicare & Medicaid Services) - PDF

National Family Caregiver Support Program (Administration on Aging)

Planning Ahead - Health, Legal, and Financial Issues From the National Institutes of Health (National Institute on Aging)

Caring for a Seriously Ill Child (Nemours Foundation)

Managing Home Health Care (For Parents) (Nemours Foundation)

Taking Care of You: Support for Caregivers (Nemours Foundation)

Caring for Kids With Medical Conditions (Nemours Foundation)

Caregiver Stress and Elder Abuse (National Center on Elder Abuse) - PDF

Caregivers' Guide to Medications and Aging (Family Caregiver Alliance)

Community-Based Care (AGS Foundation for Health in Aging)

Eldercare at Home: Caregiving (AGS Foundation for Health in Aging)

Eldercare at Home: Helping with Recovery from Illness (AGS Foundation for Health in Aging)

Eldercare at Home: Problems of Daily Living (AGS Foundation for Health in Aging)

Home Care (AGS Foundation for Health in Aging)

Patient Handouts

Bathing a patient in bed

Moving a patient from bed to a wheelchair

Pulling a patient up in bed

Turning patients over in bed

National Alliance for Caregiving

www.caregiving.org

A coalition of national organizations focused on family caregiving issues.

http://www.caregiving.org/about/about-the-alliance/

Established in 1996, the National Alliance for Caregiving is a non-profit coalition of national organizations focusing on advancing family care giving through research, innovation, and advocacy. The Alliance conducts research, does policy analysis, develops national best-practice programs, and works to increase public awareness of family care giving issues.

Our Mission: Recognizing that family caregivers provide important societal and financial contributions toward maintaining the well-being of those they care for, the Alliance is dedicated to improving quality of life for families and their care recipients through research, innovation, and advocacy.

Areas of Focus

- Caregiving Research
- Innovation and Technology
- Balanced Workplaces for Caregivers

- State & Local Caregiving Coalitions
- International Caring

http://www.caregiving.org/resources/general-caregiving/

General Caregiving: The National Alliance for Caregiving partners with other care giving associations and groups to provide additional resources to help family caregivers address and cope with the challenges of caring for a loved one.

National Family Caregiver Support Program

http://www.aoa.gov/aoa_programs/hcltc/caregiver/index.aspx or http://goo.gl/gyrWRU

The National Family Caregiver Support Program (NFCSP), established in 2000, provides grants to States and Territories, based on their share of the population aged 70 and over, to fund a range of supports that assist family and informal caregivers to care for their loved ones at home for as long as possible.

National Family Caregivers Association

www.caregiveraction.org

Information and education for family caregivers; includes the Caregiver Community Action Network, a volunteer support network in over 40 states.

National Transitions of Care Coalition

www.NTOCC.org

The last concern most individuals have when they or their loved ones are dealing with a health situation is ensuring effective communication between their doctors, nurses, social workers and other health care providers. However, poor communication between well-intentioned professionals and an expectation that patients themselves will remember and relate critical information that can lead to dangerous and even life-threatening situations. NTOCC has brought together industry leaders who have created resources to help you better understand transitional challenges and empower you as part of the care giving team.

Next Step in Care

http://www.nextstepincare.org

Next Step in Care provides easy-to-use guides to help family caregivers and health care providers work closely together to plan and implement safe and smooth transitions for chronically or seriously ill patients.

Social Security Administration

www.socialsecurity.gov

800-772-1213

Information on retirement and disability benefits, including how to sign up.

State Health Insurance Assistance Program

www.shiptalk.org

A program that offers one-on-one insurance counseling and assistance to people with Medicare and their families.

Tax deductions: how to claim caregiver tax deductions in the USA

http://www.aplaceformom.com/senior-care-resources/articles/tax-tips-for-seniors or http://goo.gl/9QORgI

The National Clearinghouse for Long-term Care Information

www.longtermcare.gov

Information and tools to plan for future long-term care needs.

Today's Caregiver

http://www.caregiver.com/

A magazine for family and professional caregivers with many resources, including a list of books for caregivers:

http://www.caregiver.com/bookclub/index.htm

Veterans Administration

(US Veterans Administration)

www.caregiver.va.gov

855-260-3274

Support and services for families caring for veterans. Maintains a VA caregiver support line.

Resources for caregivers

http://www.caregiver.va.gov/resources_landing.asp

Facebook

Here are a sampling of Facebook groups and pages. Probably the best way to find the group or page most relevant to you would be to type in "caregiver" or the name of a disease and then enter a location like Chicago, Quebec, California, Toronto.

Alzheimer's Association (679,000 likes)

Non-Profit Organization

https://www.facebook.com/actionalz/?fref=ts

Alzheimer's Awareness (509,000 likes)

Community

https://www.facebook.com/FightAlzheimers/?fref=ts

Autism Awareness (2.2 million likes)

Non-Profit Organization

https://www.facebook.com/AutismAwarenessPage/?ref=br_rs

Autism Speaks (1.5 million likes)

Charity Organization

https://www.facebook.com/autismspeaks/?fref=ts

Autism Talk (554,000 likes)

Community

https://www.facebook.com/AutismTalk/?fref=ts

Autism group (Closed group with 9300 members)

https://www.facebook.com/groups/48701140761/

Caregiver Canada

https://www.facebook.com/Caregiver-Canada-Inc-143287952402078/?fref=ts

Multiple Sclerosis International Federation (5776 likes)

Non-Profit Organization

https://www.facebook.com/MSInternationalFederation/?fref=ts

Multiple Sclerosis Foundation (15,303 members)

Public Group

https://www.facebook.com/groups/msfocus/

Multiple Sclerosis support (8385 members)

Closed Group

https://www.facebook.com/groups/202971306407870/

M.S Connect-Multiple Sclerosis (5093 members)

Closed Group

https://www.facebook.com/groups/1598134280453863/

Multiple Sclerosis Support Group (2046 likes)

Community

https://www.facebook.com/MultipleSclerosisSupportGroup/?fref=ts

National Multiple Sclerosis Society (286,000 likes)

Non-Profit Organization

https://www.facebook.com/nationalmssociety/?fref=ts

Schizophrenia (13,979 members)

Closed Group

https://www.facebook.com/groups/17300812732/

schizophrenia (6777 members)

Public Group

https://www.facebook.com/groups/2205371584/

Schizophrenia Caregiver Community (6171 likes)

Community

https://www.facebook.com/Schizophrenia24x7/?fref=ts

Google+ communities

You'll need to be logged into your Google / Gmail account to view these. Again, this is just a sampling of what's out there.

Caregiver Support and Advocacy

https://plus.google.com/u/0/communities/100659136951656
148897 (1075 members)

Caregivers

https://plus.google.com/u/0/communities/115901110758065
782410 (708 members)

Caregiver Junction

https://plus.google.com/u/0/communities/11640833861504
147311 (477 members)

Multiple Sclerosis Community

https://plus.google.com/u/0/communities/114597075829387
407446 (1471 members)

Multiple Sclerosis Support Group

https://plus.google.com/u/0/communities/109851287386479
751801 (348 members)

In recognition of World MS Day

May 27, 2015

On Monday June 15, 2015, my MS support group met for our regular monthly meeting.

We listened intently and shared our experiences over the past month in a no holds barred environment. One member shared with us a poem she received from her then young daughter written by her several years ago however, her daughter kept the poem her secret. Now an adult, married and living abroad she carefully chose the time to send the poem to her mother, May 27, World MS Day.

Here's the story: This young girl's father has MS and she is devastated. Too young to understand what is going on with the family, too afraid to find out she withdraws into her-self. Several years later she eventually left home and went far, far away overseas.

With permission from her daughter I was asked by her mom to publish the poem on my site however, the family asked to keep their identity private and I respect their request. Since I cannot duplicate content from one site to the next I invite you all to visit my site and read that sad, yet beautiful post

'A Family Almost Broken' recently published, June 16, 2015.

http://caringforcaregiver.com

The reality is that MS is a 'family' issue. It is not only the individuals inflicted with this disease that is impacted. Every family member is impacted and the children silently suffer more than we recognize.

The reluctance to talk openly about this condition hinders rather than helps families. It is a blessing that World MS Day is formed to bring public awareness about MS globally. It is healthy to talk and share. Denial is destructive and anger leads to apathy. In the end, nothing is resolved. No matter what challenges we face, together, there's strength in numbers, and, if there's a will there's a way. Be reminded you're not alone. Reach out and accept the love and support so freely offered.

What is World MS Day?

World MS Day brings the global MS community together to share stories, raise awareness and campaign with and for everyone affected by multiple sclerosis.

World MS Day is the only global awareness raising campaign for MS. Every year, the MS movement comes together to provide the public with information about MS and to raise awareness on how it affects the lives of more than 2.3 million people around the world.

Since its inception in 2009, World MS Day has grown from strength to strength, reaching hundreds of thousands of people in more than 78 countries worldwide and continuing to grow every year.

About the author

My inspiration to write this book is based on my own life experience and the many challenges navigating through a very difficult pathway. My desire to share the difficulties and rewards of care giving is to pay it forward so readers can think of the road ahead and be better prepared. Simply put, I struggled for very many years before I got a handle on my situation, I did not know what to do.

I am not a nurse, psychologist, social worker, nor do I have a designation in health services. What I do have is a wealth of practical experiences and an abundance of healthy, support of stories from caregivers in my support groups, comments on my website and caregivers whose experiences are shared. I read articles relating to care giving, books and research related topics for continuous learning.

My greatest challenge came in 1992 when care giving became my new reality. Prior to that I cared for our four children and longed for the day when I will escape care giving. Unfortunately, it was not meant to be. My husband, a detective with Toronto Police Service was diagnosed with chronic progressive multiple sclerosis in 1992. This diagnosis shattered him and devastatingly impacted our entire family. Four years after the diagnosis my husband retired from policing.

Not knowing how to deal with my new circumstances I got stronger every day navigating through whatever had to be done to keep our family going. My goal was to ensure that our children get a good education.

Thankfully, they all graduated from university and are now contributing members of society.

I became a member of the Multiple Sclerosis Society of Canada and joined a local chapter in my neighbourhood. I had to learn as much as I could about multiple sclerosis so I could understand what we were dealing with. I was on the verge of collapse, and I needed help, badly.

As I attended the meetings at the chapter I soon realized that everyone seemed to be in the same situation, carrying a tremendous stress load and had little to no communication at home, about the elephant in the room. We were all very sad, emotionally drained and broken. I knew I had to do something more for myself and for my support group.

I developed some personal friendships within the group and we spoke at length. The conversation always started off with frustration, stress, anxiety followed by tears. By the time the conversation was over there was relief, laughter and a better perspective. My friends often thanked me for listening and making them feel better

Moving forward, I decided to start a blog helping caregivers to navigate through their complex role. I trust that the information posted will impact caregivers and all readers in a positive way. Ultimately, I wish to make a difference in the lives of caregivers everywhere. We undertake a very important responsibility that is often undervalued and under appreciated.

Also, I remind caregivers that taking care of you should be your #1 priority. To be better able to take care of your loved ones, you must first take care of you.

Learn more about Author Vena Stewart-Semprie at her blog:

caringforcaregiver.com